D0415005

OLDER PEOPLE AT HOME

Older People at Home: Practical issues

Edited by

GRAHAM MULLEY
Developmental Professor of Medicine for the Elderly
Elderly Services Directorate,
St James' University Hospital,
Leeds, UK

NEIL PENN
Elderly Services Directorate,
St James' University Hospital,
Leeds, UK

EILEEN BURNS
Consultant Physician
Department for Medicine for the Elderly,
Leeds General Infirmary,
Leeds, UK

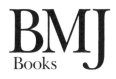

© BMJ Books 1998
BMJ Books is an imprint of the BMJ Publishing Group

All rights reserved. No part of this publication may be reproduced, stored in a retrieval system, or transmitted, in any form or by any means, electronic, mechanical, photocopying, recording and/or otherwise, without the prior written permission of the publishers.

First published in 1998
by BMJ Books, BMA House, Tavistock Square,
London WC1H 9JR

British Library Cataloguing in Publication Data

A catalogue record for this book is available from the British Library

ISBN 0-7279-1258-5

Cover image reproduced courtesy of Ulrike Preuss.

26/2/99
M

Typeset by Apek Typesetters, Nailsea, Bristol
Printed and bound by Latimer Trend, Plymouth

Contents

Editors

Eileen Burns qualified from Leeds University in 1981 and completed her general medical training in and around Leeds. She worked as a research fellow in the Department of Clinical Pharmacology at the Hallamshire Hospital in Sheffield, where she completed work on compliance and the meaurement of liver blood flow, the latter being the basis for her MD thesis. She then returned to Leeds and North and West Yorkshire, where she completed her higher medical training. In 1992 she was appointed as Consultant Geriatrician and Honorary Senior Lecturer at Leeds General Infirmary.

She has continued her interest in practical aspects affecting compliance. As she has three children under five, she has no hobbies whatsoever.

Graham Mulley qualified from Leeds Medical School in 1970. After general training in Nottingham, he spent a year as medical registrar in Nigeria, where he developed an interest in stroke research. After being MRC Research Fellow at Nottingham University where he did his doctorate on stroke, he joined Professor Tom Aire's team as Senior Registrar in Health Care of the Elderly. On returning to Leeds, he was appointed as Consultant at St James' University Hospital. In 1989 he became Developmental Professor in Elderly Medicine at Leeds University.

Professor Mulley has been Visiting Professor in San Francisco and Australia and enjoys lecturing on many aspects of geriatric medicine. His particular reseach interests are in rehabilitation, complex disability, improving the environment for disabled people and equipment for diabled older people.

He has edited two BMJ series on Aids and Appliances and received a National Consumer Plain English award for his Stroke Association booklet 'Stroke - a handbook for the patient's family'.

He is editor of *Age and Ageing*, an international scientific journal.

His spare time is spent enjoying the delights of the Yorkshire Dales and browsing in secondhand book shops.

Neil Penn qualified from Leeds Medical School in 1982. He completed his general professional training in the Yorkshire Region, obtaining the MRCP in 1985. He became Tutor in Medicine and Medicine for the Elderly in the same year and decided on a career in geriatric medicine at this time. During his time as tutor he developed a reseach interest in the relationship between nutrition, immune function and old age.

On completing his higher professional training he was appointed as a Consultant Geriatrician and Senior Clinical Lecturer at St James' University Hospital in 1992.

During any spare time he enjoys walking, fishing and reading.

Contributors

Tom Arie
Professor Emeritus
Department of Health Care of the Elderly, Medical School,
University of Nottingham, Nottingham

S Barodawala
Senior Registrar in Medicine for the Elderly
St James' University Hospital, Leeds

Mark Bradley
Consultant Physician
Department of Medicine for the Elderly, Wharfedale General
Hospital, Otley

A J Corlett
Senior Registrar in Medicine for the Elderly
St James' University Hospital, Leeds

Shah Ebrahim
Professor of Clinical Epidemiology
Department of Primary Health Care and Population Sciences,
Royal Free Hospital School of Medicine, London

Anne Forbes
Director
Catholic Agency for Social Concern, London

M Pushpangadan
Registrar
Department of Medicine for the Elderly
Leeds General Infirmary

D Renwick
Department of Medicine for the Elderly
Camborne and Redruth Hospital, Redruth, Cornwall

T A Roper
Registrar
Department of Medicine for the Elderly, St Luke's Hospital,
Bradford

Charlie Teale
Consultant Physician
Seacroft Hospital, Leeds

Anne F Travers
Senior Registrar in Public Health Medicine
South Humber Health Authority, Brigg, North Lincolnshire

P Wanklyn
Consultant Geriatrician
Leeds General Infirmary, Leeds

J Wattis
Medical Director
Leeds Community and Mental Health Trust, Leeds

John Young
Consultant Geriatrician
Bradford Hospitals Trust, St Luke's Hospital, Bradford

Foreword

Practical answers to everyday problems are not always available in textbooks. During our teaching of students and healthcare professionals, we became aware of important issues that were missing from or not well covered in journals or books. We therefore decided to focus on those topics to elderly care which were common, relevant to everyday clinical practice and which had not always been given the attention they deserved. The topics were intentionally selective - we did not try to be encyclopedic. We decided to include only a few pieces on predominantly medical subjects, as these are well described elsewhere.

The list was selected by general practitioners practising in Leeds and we are most grateful to them for telling us where problems caused them most concern or which topics needed to be demystified and made more accessible. We then drew up a list of potential contributors which included established figures and rising stars, as well as those who were just beginning to learn about the challenges and satisfactions of caring for older people.

The articles include psychological, legal, philosophical, social as well as selected medical aspects of ageing. The authors have fulfilled our expectations admirably: they have written in plain English; debunked some of the negative myths of ageing, and provided a problem-based approach to elderly care, with a particular focus on old people living at home.

The series was written primarily for general practitioners. The articles were published in the *BMJ* under the title 'Caring for Older People' and have been updated and modified in light of constructive suggestions. We have received much postive feedback not only from those in primary care but also from trainees and consultants in general medicine and old age psychiatry, as well as nurses, therapists, dietitians and social workers working with older people.

We believe that this book will be of particular help to doctors studying for the Royal College of Physicians' Diploma in Geriatric Medicine. We would like it to find a place in clinics and health centres visited by old people and on every hospital ward which admits elderly patients. We hope that copies will be read with interest and referred to frequently.

Eileen Burns
Neil D Penn
Graham P Mulley

1: Loneliness

ANNE FORBES

Loneliness is undesirable and personal: what for one person may be acceptable solitude may for another be anguish. The negative stereotype of old age includes loneliness, but the problem seriously affects only one in 10 older people. Certain people are prone to loneliness—bereaved people, immigrants, and those limited by physical disabilities—but loneliness can be exacerbated by lack of money and may occur among those in institutional care as well as older caregivers. This article discusses the signs and effects of loneliness and the schemes and activities available to support older people who may otherwise be lonely.

Loneliness may be described as an unwelcome feeling of lack or loss of companionship, or feeling that one is alone and not liking it. It is essentially undesirable and it may have implications for the health of the person experiencing it.

A situation leading to loneliness for one person can be a source of contented aloneness for someone else. Loneliness cannot be regarded as the simple, direct result of social circumstances. It is rather an individual response to an external situation to which old people vary in their reactions.

Loneliness is often confused with social isolation, a concept that can be more accurately measured (by the number of social contacts the person has, for example). However, wellbeing may not be positively correlated with social contact; much depends on the nature of the contacts made. Seeing a particular visitor may be more important than the number of people who call. For some people, solitude is a way of life which temperamentally suits them. Therefore some people may feel isolated even when they have many visitors; others who have less need of social contact may not feel lonely even if they have no visitors. This article will concentrate on loneliness, its incidence, and some suggested ways of offsetting its more disturbing effects.

How prevalent is loneliness among older people?

A report on attitudes to aging published by British Gas in 1991 found that 90% of the population (including 82% of retired people over 55) believed loneliness to be a problem associated with old age—but only 32% of the older people interviewed said that it was a problem for them personally. This bears out the findings of other American and European studies which consistently report that about two thirds of older people are never or rarely lonely; one fifth admit to being lonely sometimes, and about a tenth say that they are lonely very often.

This seems to imply on the one hand that the extent of loneliness in older people is often overestimated and on the other that it is a real problem for about one in 10 older people—almost one million people in Britain.

Which older people experience loneliness, and why?

Those most affected by loneliness are very old people, widows and widowers, and people isolated by disability. Older people who are caregivers may also be isolated and lonely. About a third of carers report feeling lonely, at least sometimes. Loneliness is more likely to occur in resident carers. Loneliness can also be experienced by older married women; older people who live with married children; those living in sheltered housing or residential care; and older people who immigrated from other countries, especially those who do not speak the language well.

Loneliness seems to be less prevalent in those rural areas where a sense of community still remains than in more densely populated urban areas. Lack of money limits the opportunities for overcoming loneliness: those on lower incomes are more prone to feelings of loneliness than those who are better off.

There is considerable debate about types of loneliness and how it is experienced by different people. Put at its simplest, there are two kinds of loneliness: external, which is brought about by the person's life circumstances (bereavement, for example) and internal, which relates more closely to personality type (Box 1.1).

What can be done?

How can we help to offset the loneliness experienced by those who are able to become involved outside the home and by those who are housebound?

Wherever possible, lonely people should be offered opportunities to reach out to others so that they retain active involvement in the

---

Box 1.1 Possible signs of loneliness

- Verbal outpouring
- Prolonged holding of one's hand or arm
- Body language:
  Defeated demeanour
  Tightly crossed arms and legs
- Drab clothing

---

pattern of their own lives, rather than sitting passively waiting for the doorbell to ring. Examples of this are given below, both for those who are able to get out and for those who are housebound. Well designed housing schemes that provide opportunities to meet others formally and informally enable lonely people to support each other. Lonely people may need encouragement and guidance on how to be creative and how to have a positive approach to meeting others.

Involvement outside the home

Community activities for all ages

Older people do not necessarily want to spend their time exclusively with other older people. There are many activities in which they can join with people of other ages:

- Adult education classes—for example, painting, creative writing
- Involvement in community action—for example, membership of Good Neighbour schemes, which visit housebound people; local history groups; sporting activities such as bowling
- Membership of local churches
- Participation in locally organised outings, either to the country-side or to the theatre or cinema; holidays.

To facilitate the involvement of older people, however active, it is helpful if clear information is available well in advance, transport is provided if necessary, and meetings are organised at a suitable time (preferably during daylight hours) in a warm comfortable venue with good seating.

Details of local community activities can be obtained from the local Council for Voluntary Service (whose number will be found in the telephone book) or from the local library or possibly the social services area office. Councils for Voluntary Service are usually considered the de facto headquarters or liaison point for voluntary groups in the city or district. Information about church activities may be available from the local Churches Together group.

Activities with other older people

In addition to many of the suggestions above, activities with other older people include the following:

- The University of the Third Age (UTA, Head Office, 26 Harrison Street, London WC1H 8JG (tel 0171 837 8838)) offers locally run courses (not necessarily academic); no qualifications are needed, no diplomas are awarded, and many of the teachers are retired people
- Smaller gatherings of three or four people who share an interest—for example, gardening, sport, Bible study—who are invited into the home of a younger person for coffee or afternoon tea. One national group encouraging schemes whereby people are invited for afternoon tea, etc, is Contact (15 Henrietta Street, London WC2E 8QH (tel 0171 240 0630, fax 0171 379 5781)); it will supply names of leaders of local groups
- Luncheon clubs are run both by voluntary organisations (such as church groups, Age Concern) and by the social services department of local authorities; they offer social activity as well as a hot meal
- Reminiscence and local history groups can be very stimulating if they are well and sensitively run; the social services area office or Age Concern can usually supply details
- Holidays for older people are organised by Saga Holidays (Bouverie House, Middelburg Square, Folkestone, Kent CT20 1AZ (tel 0800 300 456)).

Specialist groups

Certain specialist groups may be of assistance at times of loss, either through bereavement, retirement, or illness:

- Cruse—named after the container of oil belonging to a biblical widow—offers counselling and support after bereavement. Local groups, established around the country, offer a drop–in centre, a telephone advisory line, literature, and individual visits by trained counsellors; details of local groups are available from 126 Sheen Road, Richmond, Surrey TW9 1UR (tel 0181 940 4818). Cruse also operates a Bereavement Line offering counselling to bereaved people (tel 0181 332 7227).

• Support groups for people with a particular illness can be helpful—for example, the Parkinson's Disease Society, Arthritis Care, the Stroke Association, and the Alzheimer's Disease Society.

Suggestions for housebound people

Ways of bringing more people into the house

Most areas have befriending schemes, which can be very supportive provided that clear boundaries are set and the "befrienders" know what is and is not expected of them. Contact them through the local Age Concern group, local churches (in some areas the Methodist church has "live at home" schemes), or community care schemes linked to the area office of the social services department.

Ways in which housebound people can feel useful to others

One way that housebound people can feel useful is through offering telephone support to others who are isolated, such as carers or other older housebound people. In one neighbourhood a telephone circle was established, in which seven housebound people each rang one of the group each morning to ensure they were well. If help was needed, a contact person was available. Another useful activity is letter writing, perhaps for a worthy cause (such as Amnesty International) or corresponding with a pen pal.

Getting a telephone

A telephone not only gives the reassurance of being able to request help in an emergency, but also allows the opportunity to chat to friends and family. Some local authorities offer financial help with installation costs.

Housing provision and loneliness

Suitable housing can play a significant part in alleviating loneliness. There is a range of provisions which can help: central alarm systems; contact with a warden; well designed, resident friendly buildings; and care and repair schemes.

One organisation, the Abbeyfield Society (Abbeyfield House, 53

5

Box 1.2   Practice points

- Consider loneliness in any isolated older person—especially housebound people, those who fall, those with impaired mobility or sensory impairment, bereaved people, and those with dementia
- Lonely people who are reluctant to go out may be troubled by depression, agoraphobia, deafness, or urinary incontinence, all of which might respond to treatment
- Alcoholism and depression may be exacerbated through lack of company
- Lonely and isolated old people are at risk of nutritional problems, which should be considered
- As well as receiving visitors and telephone calls and going on outings, lonely old people may be helped by becoming pet owners

---

Victoria Street, St Albans, Herts AL1 3UW (tel 01727 857536)), which is particularly aware of the loneliness of many older people, has developed family style houses where older people can live together with care and companionship.

Conclusion

Although most older people do not experience loneliness, there is evidence that for about one in three people this can be a problem. For the 10% seriously affected, loneliness may have a detrimental effect on their health.

General practitioners and community nurses are in a unique position to identify loneliness as they are in contact with very old people, bereaved people, and people with disabilities—the three groups most at risk. If they were to encourage some of the initiatives mentioned here, as many do, much of the distress of loneliness might be eased (Box 1.2).

Recommended reading

Marriott V, Timbick T. *Loneliness: how to overcome it.* London: Age Concern England, 1988. (This gives useful advice and a directory of helpful organisations and is available from Age Concern England, 1268 London Road, London SW16 4EJ (tel 0181 679 8000)).

2: Elder abuse

MARK BRADLEY

Elder abuse takes many forms and occurs in a variety of settings; it is both under-recognised and under-reported. Despite a lack of statutory guidelines or legislation, effective management is possible. More could be done to recognise abuse, and healthcare workers need to be vigilant, paying attention to both the circumstances in which abuse occurs and its warning signs. Elder abuse may be physical, sexual, psychological, or financial. It may be intentional, unintentional, or the result of neglect. It causes harm to the older person either temporarily or over a period of time. The often quoted stereotype of a highly dependent white woman over the age of 75 who is being physically abused by her son or daughter is only a small aspect of this problem. The scale of the problem is not known as there is no accepted way of recording cases. Attention is increasingly being focused on elder abuse, largely because of the influence of the Community Care Act. Many cases, however, go unreported.

Background

There are many reasons why older people are abused. The most common include deteriorating family relationships, caregivers who have been abused themselves, social isolation, psychopathology of the abuser, and imbalance of power between abused and abuser. Caring for a sick, dependent elderly person is a challenge for even the most capable person. When caregivers to older people have little support from within the community they may suffer intolerable strain and this may lead to elder abuse. Disturbed sleep, difficult behaviour, and faecal incontinence often result in severe strain on the caregiver and may set the scene for abuse. Many caregivers express feelings of frustration, despair, anxiety and of not being cared for themselves. They often feel that the situation is beyond their control. Difficult situations are often compounded by strained family relationships where, for instance, a son or daughter feels a duty to care for a parent of whom they have never been particularly fond or who has treated them badly in the past. The abuser, of course, may be a spouse rather than a younger member

7

of the family. The excessive personal use of alcohol or tranquillising drugs by caregivers can have a disinhibiting effect, which may lead to emotions being translated into physical actions.

Physical abuse is the most commonly encountered form of elder abuse as it is the most easily recognised. Financial abuse, neglect, and sexual abuse are probably both under-recognised and under-reported. Psychological abuse in the form of aggression, humiliation, and intimidation is the most difficult to identify and quantify (Box 2.1).

Intervention

Intervention is complicated and should always be interdisciplinary. There is no correct way of managing elder abuse. It is seldom appropriate for only one person or agency to tackle the problem. Effective intervention will probably involve local authority social services, the health authority, police, and private and voluntary

---

Box 2.1 Warning signs

Background of abuse
- Poor family relationships
- History of family violence
- Low income, perhaps with inadequate housing
- Caregivers who are emotionally, physically, and socially isolated
- Lack of privacy for caregivers
- Frequent calls to local agencies
- History of alcohol or drug abuse or mental illness in caregivers

Suspicious circumstances
- Unexplained falls, burns, and fractures
- Bruises in unusual places, such as the inside of the thigh; pinchmarks on the arms
- Inappropriate administration of medication by caregivers
- Provision of inappropriate clothing
- Being left in wet clothing

Signs of financial abuse
- Unexpected inability to pay bills
- Disparity between assets and living conditions

Signs of sexual abuse
- Overt sexual behaviour
- Torn or stained underclothes
- Genital infection and irritation
- "Love" bites
- Bruising and lacerations in the rectovaginal area

---

agencies. These agencies should have policies and guidelines for dealing with suspected cases of elder abuse, along with support and training, but often there is no clear framework within which to work. In Britain there is no formalised procedure for dealing with elder abuse, unlike much of the United States, where specific legislation and protocols exist.

A sequence of identification, assessment, and action is usually followed.

Identification is usually through the warning signs given in the box. Warning signs could be spotted by anyone, professional or otherwise, caring for an older person.

Assessment should be done by an interdisciplinary team, which should assess both the caregiver and the patient, focusing on the suspected abuse and its likely cause. A more extensive care planning meeting may be required for complex cases.

Action will result in provision of a care package designed to deal specifically with the situation, ideally allowing the abused person to remain in their own home.

All cases of proved or suspected abuse should be kept under regular review.

Clearly the final care package will vary from case to case but is likely to include some of the following: health information and support, respite care, day care, home care including nursing, provision of aids and appliances, continence advice, financial advice, advocacy, legal or police intervention, rehousing, and institutional care. Removal of an older person from their home should be seen as a last resort and should not be done without their consent. Support services that are provided should aim to deal with specific problems and should not simply be offered in an attempt "to do something." It should be remembered that most cases of abuse are due to caregiver stress and that intervention will often need to be aimed at helping caregivers to overcome the problems that they themselves are facing. Most caregivers would wish to care in a loving and sensitive way. (Boxes 2.2 to 2.4 for case examples.)

Legislation

Britain has no clear legal framework designed to deal specifically with elder abuse, but there is however some legislation that may be used in certain circumstances. Criminal legislation is seldom useful as the victims of abuse are often afraid and unable to give sufficient

Box 2.2   The case of Mr C

Mr C, a retired miner living at home, is admitted to hospital because of deteriorating mobility and falls. After rehabilitation and treatment for pseudogout and gait apraxia he returns home with increased support from social services. Unfortunately he is readmitted two weeks later with further falls. He feels that he can no longer manage at home and asks the hospital social worker about going into residential care. His son has been "looking after" his financial affairs, collecting his state and occupational pensions and using them to pay the bills. Mr C has little idea what happens to the rest of his money and cannot understand why his son refuses to cooperate with the social services' financial assessment and why he never visits him in hospital.

evidence to secure conviction in a court. The victim often denies the abuse.

National Assistance Act

Section 47 of the National Assistance Act 1948 allows a local authority with the certificate of a community physician to apply to a magistrate for removal of the elderly person from their home to a place of safety if the person concerned is suffering from a grave chronic disease or, being aged, infirm, or incapacitated, is living in insanitary conditions; the person is unable to give himself or herself proper care and attention; or the person's removal from home is necessary in their best interests or for preventing injury or serious nuisance to other people. A 1951 amendment allows for the

Box 2.3   The case of Mrs D

Mrs D lives alone in rented accommodation. Despite a previous stroke, she is reasonably independent in her flat, relying on her family only to collect her pension and to do some shopping. Over a short period of time she becomes increasingly unwell and relies more heavily on her family, but after successful inpatient treatment for a chest infection she returns to her former largely independent self. After a successful home visit she is looking forward to returning to her flat. Over the next few days she becomes more withdrawn, and then suddenly announces that she has decided that she should "go into a home." Subsequent questioning reveals that family members have visited and made it clear that they believe she should not return home; they have threatened that unless she goes "into a home" they will have nothing more to do with her.

Box 2.4   The case of Mrs E

Mrs E, an elderly Asian woman, lives with her son and his children. She sleeps downstairs, is mobile only with a Zimmer frame, and is occasionally incontinent. She has had a fractured femur and also a fractured humerus. She is admitted to hospital with a painful knee and immobility. Radiographs reveal a fracture of the proximal tibia. She tells an Asian hospital worker that her granddaughter shouts at her when she is incontinent and has kicked her. She does not want to return home. When seen later by an Asian social worker she denies the earlier claims, saying she has slipped. It becomes clear, however, that most of her care at home is provided not by her son and his wife but by the young teenage granddaughter. She continues to deny any further abuse and asks to return home. The family declines all offers of any further help and denies that Mrs E has been kicked. Her son feels that it is his duty to look after his mother. Mrs E is discharged home to be monitored by social services, her general practitioner, and the district nurse.

---

removal without delay of a person for up to three weeks on the application of the community physician supported by a second medical opinion.

Community Care Act

Section 47 of the Community Care Act 1990 requires local authorities to carry out assessments of need where people appear to them to be in need of services.

Mental Health Act

Under the Mental Health Act 1983 the local authority or an individual may be appointed guardian to a person who is mentally ill. This lasts for six months and there is a right of appeal. Section 115 allows an approved social worker to enter and inspect premises in which a mentally disordered patient is living if he or she has cause to believe that the patient is not under proper care. Section 127(2) provides that it is an offence for an individual to wilfully neglect a mentally ill person in his or her guardianship. Section 135 allows for a person to be removed to a place of safety for up to 72 hours.

Court of Protection

The Court of Protection has jurisdiction when a person is incapable by reason of mental disorder of managing and admin-

11

Box 2.5

The Elder Abuse Response Line—0800 731 4141—takes calls from older people, carers, and professionals concerned about elder abuse. It is available Monday to Friday 10 am to 4.30 pm. This is a multilingual service. Action on Elder Abuse are available for more general enquiries (including membership) at: AEA, Astral House, 1268 London Road, London SW16 4ER (tel 0181 764 7648).

---

istering his or her property and affairs. The court has wide powers relating to property and affairs but not to matters relating directly to a person's care. A receiver is usually appointed; this is often a relative but it can be anyone suitable. The receiver is not allowed to dispose of assets.

Power of attorney

Power of attorney allows a person to give authority, for financial matters, to someone else to act on his or her behalf. Enduring power of attorney is initiated while the person is of sound mind and continues when he or she becomes mentally incapable.

Suggested reading

Age Concern, British Geriatrics Society, Carers National Association, Help the Aged, Police Federation. *Abuse of elderly people. Guidelines for action.* London: Age Concern England, 1990.

Department of Health, Social Services Inspectorate. *No longer afraid. The safeguard of older people in domestic settings.* London: HMSO, 1993.

Social Services Inspectorate. *Confronting elder abuse.* London: HMSO, 1992.

3: Ethnic elders

SHAH EBRAHIM

The numbers of elderly people from ethnic groups within Britain is rising rapidly as postwar immigrants age. Ethnic elders face problems owing to age-associated increased risks of common chronic diseases, racial discrimination, and poor access to many health services and social services. This disadvantage will be alleviated through increased understanding of health beliefs held by ethnic elders and ensuring better access to services through mechanisms such as employment of more staff from ethnic minority groups in senior positions, better training of staff, and more appropriate and sensitive environments. The myths that family care is sufficient, that no use of services implies no need, and that assimilation into the majority population will occur must be discounted.

Since the 1870s Britain has received large numbers of immigrants from different countries and cultures (Fig. 3.1). Migration is due to "push" and "pull" factors. After the second world war, Britain actively recruited labour from Commonwealth countries to aid the reconstruction effort—a major "pull"; many came thinking

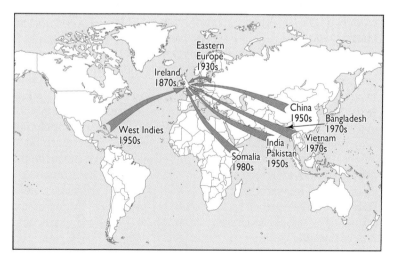

Figure 3.1   Trends in world migration to Britain

13

Box 3.1   OPCS classification of ethnicity for 1991 census

White	Pakistani
Black—Caribbean	Bangladeshi
Black—African	Chinese
Black—other	Asian—other
Indian	Other

they would earn enough money to return home and retire in comfort. "Push" factors are poverty, political instability, and oppression.

Immigration policy became much less flexible during the 1980s and led to reductions in the numbers of new arrivals. New migrants arrive daily from some countries (such as Somalia) where political oppression endangers life but not from others (former Yugoslavia). British immigration policies are not consistent (Box 3.1).

It is still possible for older people from some countries to resettle in Britain by joining their children. The distribution of ethnic minorities in Britain is strongly biased towards inner city areas of major industrial towns. Bradford, Leeds, Manchester, Nottingham, Wolverhampton, Leicester, Birmingham, Coventry, and London have high numbers of elderly people of different ethnic origins.

Ethnicity

Ethnicity is a complex idea. It includes skin colour, culture, language, religion, birth place, food, beliefs, and behaviour. Ethnicity is impossible to define clearly and in most contexts refers to the "otherness" of people who do not belong to the predominant population. The classification used by the Office of Population Censuses and Surveys[1] emphasises the "visible" criterion of skin colour, reflecting British views of ethnicity. Not surprisingly, people who share a skin colour do not necessarily have much else in common. It is wrong to assume that people of the same colour should be put together as they will "get on better." Many of the problems of ethnic elders are common to European, Irish, and other "invisible" groups.

The numbers of people belonging to different ethnic groups are relatively small—about 5% overall. Most people from ethnic

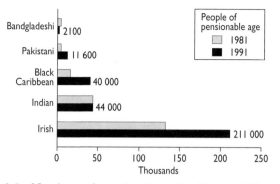

Figure 3.2 Numbers of people of pensionable age (60 and over for women, 65 and over for men) identified from 1981 and 1991 censuses

minorities in Britain are young compared with white British people; only 5-10% of people of other ethnic origin are over 65 years old.

All the populations of people who arrived in Britain in the 1950s and 1960s in their 20s and 30s are aging rapidly and reaching retirement (Fig. 3.2). The numbers of older people from ethnic minorities will increase dramatically over the next two decades.

Jeopardy

Ethnic elders are at risk by virtue of old age because of associated ill health and loss of role. They are further jeopardised by the multiple disadvantages due to racism, resulting in poor living conditions, overcrowding, low incomes, and a sense of alienation. They do not make use of many statutory and voluntary services because they perceive these services as being for the majority white population and being insensitive to their needs.[2]

Disease patterns are broadly a reflection of those experienced by most older people. Rare or "exotic" tropical diseases are seldom encountered, but the diagnosis of heart failure, asthma, or tuberculosis may present a major challenge because of communication problems. With the exception of Chinese people, older people from all ethnic groups seem to have more chronic disease than white British people until very old age (Fig. 3.3).[1] Explanations for the excess morbidity are poverty, poor housing, and lifestyle (smoking, lack of exercise, diet), all of which contribute to higher risks of cardiovascular disease, diabetes, and other chronic

15

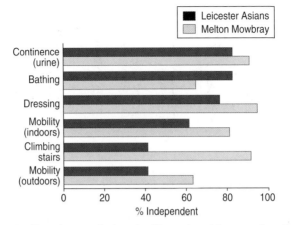

Figure 3.3 Prevalence of chronic illness in older people of different ethnic groups, 1991 census

problems. Morbidity may be due to factors operating in the "home" country, selection of who migrates, or the process of adaptation and adjustment (Box 3.2).[3]

Health beliefs

A variety of beliefs can determine our views about causation and treatment of disease. Many older people from ethnic minorities (in common with many white British people) hold contradictory beliefs, ranging from a modern understanding of infectious and chronic degenerative disease, a religious view that it is God's will that disease occurs and that prayer will help, and traditional beliefs in spirits or the "evil eye" that must be dealt with by rituals.

It is not possible to generalise about the specific beliefs held by an individual. Sensitive inquiry about beliefs should be an essential part of taking a history, whatever the patient's ethnicity.

Box 3.2   Triple jeopardy for ethnic elders

- Age
- Cultural and racial discrimination
- Lack of access to health, housing, and social services

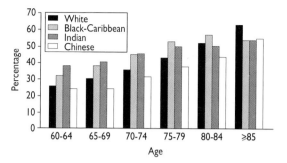

Figure 3.4 General practice consultations of Asians in inner Leicester compared with Melton Mowbray (predominantly white population)

Consultations in primary care

The number of consultations in general practice by older people from ethnic minorities is high (Fig. 3.4),[4] and this may cause consternation for the general practitioner or nurse (Box 3.3). Having excluded anaemia, osteomalacia, tuberculosis, diabetes, asthma, and ischaemic heart disease, what next? Most older people from ethnic minorities consider themselves to be sicker than white British people. This suggests that excess consultation may simply reflect excess ill health.

Non-specific symptoms are common, and ethnic elders with "modern" health beliefs may expect a suitable array of strong medicines (even injections) to deal with them.

The general practitioner must be aware that these patients are likely to have multiple consultations with alternative practitioners and to take drugs obtained overseas, and should ask about these practices. Employing practice staff from a predominant local ethnic minority group is an excellent way of gaining insight into these expectations and practices.

Box 3.3   Common diseases among ethnic elders

- Ischaemic heart disease
- Stroke
- Diabetes
- Asthma
- Tuberculosis
- Osteomalacia
- Cataract
- "Exotica"—tropical diseases

The hospital experience

Hospital admission is a frightening, demeaning, and difficult experience for anyone and is even harder for ethnic elders. Familiarity with hospital routines (which white people gain from watching TV hospital soaps) is non-existent, and language may present insuperable barriers. Staff from ethnic minorities can help make hospitals more sensitive to people's needs. However, it is vital that equal employment opportunities are not limited to menial roles if improvements in equity and accessibility of services are to be achieved (Box 3.4).

Rehabilitation

The process of rehabilitation is not widely understood by many ethnic elders. If you are ill, you should lie in bed until you get better or die. Active rehabilitation may be thought unhelpful and is counterintuitive. Careful explanation and negotiation is required with the patient and family and with community services to establish aims and methods of rehabilitation and to ensure a reasonable outcome.[5]

Activities of daily living are widely used to assess progress and determine discharge from hospital and the need for follow up rehabilitation. Aims are culturally specific and differences in customs of dressing, bathing, and eating must be taken into account. These factors may explain some, but not all, of the relative dependency of Asians aged over 75 in Leicester (Fig. 3.5).[4]

Language, religion, and food are the most obvious differences between ethnic groups, but the health service and social services are not responding to these needs in ways that reflect our

---

Box 3.4   Creating a better hospital environment

Interpreters—available for inpatient and outpatient work
Meals—culturally appropriate and likely to be enjoyed by all
Visiting—acceptance of large family groups, particularly after death
Signs—use of direction markings comprehensible to those not literate in any language
Patient information—booklets, cassette tapes, hospital radio in several languages
Discharge and follow up—equity with white population in provision
Equal opportunities employment at all levels—ethnic monitoring, particularly of medical shortlisting and appointments committees

---

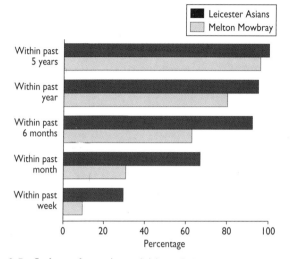

Figure 3.5 Independence in activities of daily living among Asians in inner Leicester and white people in Melton Mowbray

multicultural society. Provision of trained interpreters, places for prayer, and culturally acceptable food are all needed in hospitals but are seldom found.

Religious beliefs and social customs must be observed to ensure that the processes of dying and bereavement are not made unnecessarily painful. Knowledge of practices of the major religions (Box 3.5) is not widespread. It is always sensible to ask relatives about specific requirements and not to make assumptions.

Family and social factors

The return home in old age was the expectation of many migrants, particularly from the West Indies. For many this hope will never be realised, but some may have the resources and desire to bury their bones on home soil. Arranging for overseas travel for a frail or very dependent person is quite possible and can often result in much happiness. It is vital that the family have clear information to give the airline on the person's disabilities and likely needs during travel. A comprehensive medical, nursing, and treatment summary is also essential for continuity of care once the person gets back home.

The social services have made little progress in adapting to our

19

Box 3.5   Death rituals in different cultures

Judaism—Lay out body conventionally; wrap in plain sheet with no religious emblems. Body should not be left alone. Burial within 24 hours. Postmortem examination only in exceptional cases
Sikhism—Belief in reincarnation. Family may wish to wash and dress the body. Cremation within 24 hours. White worn as a sign of mourning
Hinduism—A Hindu priest (pandit) will arrange cremation with variable rituals. Open expression of grief is expected. Postmortem examination is felt to be disrespectful to the deceased
Islam[6]— Relatives are duty bound to visit the bereaved. Running water is needed for washing before prayers. Family usually carry out rites but local mosque will help. Body should be touched only by Muslims; non-Muslims should wear disposable gloves when touching the body. Burial should be done within 24 hours
Buddhism—Belief in reincarnation. Cremation arranged at an auspicious time determined by monks. No fundamental objections to postmortem examination
Christianity—Family usually wish to see and may watch over the body. Last rites may be arranged by priest before death. Cremation or burial depending on preference. No fundamental objections to postmortem examination

---

multicultural society.[7] This is a reflection of political pressure to sustain services for the white (voting) majority, assumptions that no use equals no need, and a widely held belief that assimilation into the wider population will occur (see Box 3.6). Thus the need for specific ethnic services is avoided. In general, social services should now be making contracts for service provision of meals on wheels, home care, day centres, and lunch clubs with local voluntary groups run by ethnic minorities themselves.

The extended family is popularly believed to exist among ethnic minorities and to be capable of coping with almost any chronic disease. Extended family groups work by mutual support through well defined roles. A dementing older person is not able to fulfil a

---

Box 3.6   Myths about ethnic elders

- Numbers are very small
- The family supports old people
- No use of services equals no need for services
- People from ethnic minorities will return home in old age
- It would be better if they spoke English

---

useful role, and supervision and care become major problems when everyone else is out at school and work. To cope successfully, families require advice, support, respite, and practical help with disability and financial benefits.

References

1 Office of Population Censuses and Surveys. *Census for Great Britain, 1991.* London: HMSO, 1991.
2 Norman A. *Triple jeopardy: growing old in a second homeland.* London: Centre for Policy on Ageing, 1985.
3 Marmot M, Adelstein AM, Bulusi L. *Immigrant mortality in England and Wales (1970-78): causes of death by country.* London: HMSO, 1984. (OPCS studies of medical and population subjects 47.)
4 Donaldson L. Health and social status of elderly Asians: a community survey. *BMJ* 1986;**293**:1079-82.
5 Squires AJ, ed. *Multicultural health care and rehabilitation of older people.* London: Edward Arnold, 1991.
6 Gatrad AR. Muslim customs surrounding death, bereavement, postmortem examinations, and organ transplants. *BMJ* 1994;**309**:521-3.
7 Morton J, ed. *Recent research on services for black and minority ethnic elderly people.* London: Age Concern, Institute of Gerontology, 1993. (Ageing Update.)

SCHOOL OF MEDICINE & DENTISTRY LIBRARY
ST. BARTHOLOMEW'S HOSPITAL

4: Some legal aspects of mental capacity

TOM ARIE

This chapter discusses some practical matters which arise when competence to make decisions is in question. Consent, testamentary capacity, powers of attorney, the Court of Protection, "living wills," and research on people with dementia are briefly considered.

Doctors and other health workers are often asked for an opinion on the capacity of an older person to make a decision or give a signature. These decisions can be difficult, for there are "grey areas" and there may often be uncertainty. The principles for assessing testamentary capacity will often be helpful; they clarify other similar questions of competence.

Testamentary capacity

Testamentary capacity requires that the subject should understand the nature of the act being undertaken—that a will is being made and what a will is. The person should have a reasonable awareness of the nature and extent of the assets to be distributed and should be aware of who might reasonably have a claim to be considered as beneficiaries of the will. Judgment must not be clouded by delusions or other significant mental illness.

Practical points

- Though the person must know that he or she is making a will, and what a will is, it is not essential to know the exact value, say, of a house that will form part of the estate. However, not to know that there is a house would normally be a significant deficiency.
- A person is not bound to leave his or her money to anyone in particular, but a will would clearly be invalid if the person making it had forgotten that he or she was married, or the existence of some or all of the children.
- It is usually acceptable for judgment to be influenced by likes or dislikes, but not by psychotic ideas.

Determining capacity

When a doctor or other health worker is asked for an opinion on mental capacity, the basis for the opinion—whether negative or positive—must always be clearly recorded. The facts may later be challenged. Careful and searching questions must be asked: it is not enough to record a conclusion. Simple standard tests of cognitive function are usually desirable.

Many people who are grossly mentally impaired may long preserve a deceptively reassuring social facade.

A person who is in hospital on account of mental disorder should never sign any document without the knowledge of the doctor in charge. This rule (which should be universal in psychiatric units) should be included in ward information booklets given to patients and relatives. This applies also to mentally incapacitated people in nursing homes or similar settings.

Consent to treatment

When obtaining consent to treatment, the doctor's overriding concern must always be to do what is in the patient's best interests. Every attempt should be made to ensure that the patient understands the nature of the treatment and its risks and benefits—this may require the use of large print and clear wording on forms and patience on the part of whoever is explaining.

Forgetfulness may sometimes have little bearing on ability to understand. Older people have the same rights to self determination as those who are younger (Box 4.1).

Power of attorney

Power of attorney is a legal document whereby one person (the donor) enables another person of his or her choice (the attorney) to act on his or her behalf. The attorney can then act as if he or she were the donor.

To give a valid power of attorney the donor must pass essentially the same tests as those for testamentary capacity. The power may be limited to specific acts (for example, selling the house) or it may be "general," covering all financial matters.

In English law an ordinary power of attorney—made when the donor is mentally well—automatically ceases to be valid if he or she becomes mentally incompetent.

Box 4.1   Practical points—consent to treatment

- Questions of treatment should always be discussed with the relatives of a mentally incapacitated person, but their relationship does not give legal authority to make decisions on the patient's behalf
- When there are uncertainties about the patient's competence, it is wise to consult other colleagues who know the patient, or to get independent opinions from those who don't. It may be appropriate to obtain the opinion of a psychiatrist or psychogeriatrician on the patient's mental state
- Confusion may be transient, and mild dementia may not be incompatible with ability to give informed consent
- A patient's lack of objection is often taken as consent ("the not unwilling patient"), but even this has been challenged

---

Enduring power of attorney

Since an ordinary power of attorney lapses if the donor becomes mentally incompetent, many countries have introduced the enduring power of attorney. This provides that, should the donor become mentally incapable, the power continues to have effect.

England and Wales introduced enduring power of attorney in 1985; in Scotland an ordinary power of attorney signed after 1 January 1991 remains valid even if the donor loses capacity, unless the original document specifies otherwise. Before the enduring power of attorney was instituted, it was necessary to make over the affairs of a person who became mentally incompetent to the Court of Protection (see below). This could be costly and time consuming.

Like an ordinary power of attorney, an enduring power of attorney is restricted to financial matters: it does not cover decisions on medical treatment or non-financial personal arrangements. It can refer to specific acts or can be "general."

The donor can require the enduring power of attorney to take effect at once and continue despite subsequent incapacity; or to take effect only if the donor should become incompetent.

The enduring power of attorney must be made on a prescribed form which is available from stationers. The form must be signed by the donor, the attorney, and a witness (who does not need to be a professional person, though doctors are quite often asked to be witnesses). If competence is in question, it may be sensible to ask a psychiatrist (or psychogeriatrician) to be a witness. Like a will, an enduring power of attorney can be made without the help of a solicitor. But it is in practice wise to ask a solicitor to ensure that the form has been correctly completed.

The donor may appoint one or more attorneys to act either jointly or "severally" (that is, each may act alone). Having two attorneys is a good idea since one or other may be unavailable (or no longer alive) when they come to be needed; and having two to act jointly gives "checks and balances," if these are felt to be necessary. However, if attorneys have to act jointly, the power of attorney lapses if one of them dies. Generally, people choose their spouse and a child or close relative or solicitor as their attorneys.

If the attorney believes that the donor has become mentally incapable, the enduring power of attorney must be registered with the Court of Protection (there is a fee). The donor and certain stipulated close relatives must then be informed and have the right to object. The Court of Protection can terminate the enduring power of attorney if, for instance, the appointed attorney has become mentally incapable or is found to be dishonest. The Court of Protection does not routinely supervise the attorney after an enduring power of attorney has been registered—but it may do so if it feels it necessary.

The attorney has limited powers to benefit himself or herself from the donor's assets—for example, if the donor's attorney is a child to whom the donor has been in the habit of giving an annual gift exempt from inheritance tax he or she may continue to take that sum, on the basis that the donor would have wished to continue to give it (Box 4.2).

The Court of Protection

The Court of Protection exists to supervise the management of the affairs of those (known as "patients" of the court) who are mentally incapable of doing so themselves. The Court's powers relate only to financial matters. The court can write a will for an incapacitated person, either when no will exists, or to supersede an existing will which is no longer appropriate.

Referral to the Court of Protection should be considered:

- When it is believed (by a relative, friend, doctor, social worker, or other key person) that the patient is not capable of managing his or her affairs because of mental incapacity, and when bank accounts and property are not held in joint names with another person—and when there is no enduring power of attorney;

Box 4.2   Practical points—enduring power of attorney

- It has been established in the courts that the mere existence of a degree of dementia does not preclude the making of an enduring power of attorney, provided the necessary criteria can still be reasonably met
- An enduring power of attorney should always be considered in the early stages of a dementing, or potentially dementing, illness
- It may be sensible for entirely well people to make an enduring power of attorney, just as it is sensible to make a will—a road traffic accident may happen tomorrow. The enduring power of attorney may never need to be used, but it gives the reassurance that, should incapacity occur, one's affairs will be managed by someone whom one has chosen

---

- When the patient's financial state justifies it: for those with limited assets (say, a total estate of less than £5000) "Directions of the Public Trustee" can be sought (this can be useful in arranging payment, for instance, of nursing home fees); for small matters, like drawing of a state pension, arrangements can usually be made with the social security authorities without recourse to the Court of Protection;
- When there is dispute, among the family perhaps, as to who should handle the patient's financial affairs; if there are no relatives; or if it is thought that someone may be dealing dishonestly with the patient's affairs.

Usually the nearest relative applies to the court, but anyone with a legitimate interest may apply. Personal referral is possible, but it is usually done through a solicitor. A Citizens' Advice Bureau may give helpful advice.

The doctor's role in referrals to the Court of Protection is to complete a medical certificate stating that the patient is incapable of managing his or her affairs by virtue of a mental disorder, the nature of which must be described. A fee can be charged.

The court's procedures

The court charges a commencement fee, an annual administration fee (which varies with the patient's income), and a fee for any major transaction which the court may authorise (such as selling a house). Fees may run to hundreds of pounds, or more, in some cases.

The court will require details of the patient's assets and financial commitments and will make an enquiry into all circumstances. If assets are small, "Directions of the Public Trustee" can be issued usually within weeks.

For those with larger assets, the court appoints a "receiver." This misleading term means an "administrator" who is appointed to manage the patient's affairs under the supervision of the court. Usually this is a close relative or a solicitor or accountant. In Scotland a curator bonis is appointed on application to the Court of Session.

The receiver is authorised to draw on the patient's money for clothing and personal needs up to an agreed maximum. Receivers must ensure that the patient receives all social security entitlements, that any property is kept in good order, that buildings are insured, and tax affairs dealt with. They can apply to use capital to pay for nursing home or similar care or to maintain the patient at home. They can also apply for special authority to make loans and investments on the patient's behalf or to buy a piece of special equipment or furniture for the patient's benefit.

Living wills (advance directives)

Powers of attorney and the Court of Protection deal only with material assets. Living wills are concerned with decisions about treatment, especially at the end of life. A person in sound mind might stipulate that, should he or she become incapable of decisions and develop particular grievous illnesses, then certain treatments should, or should not, be given.

In England and Wales advance refusal of treatment generally has force in common law, and other advance directives have moral force in issues such as relief of pain. Views of relatives, close friends, or appointed attorneys carry moral force if they are based on evidence of what the likely wishes would have been when the patient was well.

Various drafts of advance directives are available, and an excellent book considers the subject in detail (see below).

Research

Questions of consent to research on severely demented people (as on children) remain problematic. Again, consent of close

27

Box 4.3   Practical points

- "Advance directives" have no formal place in English law, but are part of the current agenda of active debate. In the absence of precise legal provision, the doctor must, as in all things, be seen to act in good faith, taking into account any evidence of what the patient would have wished had he or she had the capacity validly to indicate this.
- The Alzheimer's Disease Society now has an agreement with Lawnet, a group of solicitors who offer a named person specialising in the type of advice carers need. There is a fee, but people referred by the Society may receive an initial half hour consultation free of charge.

---

relatives is always desirable, but has no legal force. Ethics committees understandably find these issues difficult.

In December 1997 the Government issued a consultation document ('green paper'): *Who Decides? Making Decisions on behalf of mentally incapacitated adult*. This proposes wide changes in legislation in England and Wales, based on proposals from the Law Commission. These might include provision for a 'general power to act reasonably' on behalf of an incapacitated person, and a 'continuing power of atorney' which could extend also to decisions other than financial. Thus whilst at present the position remains as described in this chapter, it may in many respects change.

Further information

The Public Trust Office (Protection Division, Stewart House, 24 Kingsway, London WC2B 6JX (tel 0171 664 7300)) makes available a *Handbook for Receivers* and a booklet of *Guidance on Enduring Powers of Attorney*. Similarly, the Accountant of Court, Parliament House, Edinburgh EH1 1RF (tel 0131 225 2595) in Scotland provides a booklet of *Information for Families of Persons Subject to Curatory*.

A detailed consideration of "living wills" is given in *Let Me Decide: The Health Care Directive that Speaks For You When You Can't* by W Molloy and V Mepham, published by Penguin in 1993.

5: What an old age psychiatrist does

J WATTIS

Mental illness is common in old age and is also often associated with physical illness and social problems, whether these be general deprivation or traumatic life events. Its detection demands vigilance and its diagnosis and management demand teamwork. This chapter considers three major disorders, but other problems such as drug and alcohol dependence and schizophrenia do occur, though they are mercifully rare compared with depression, delirium, and dementia.

Old age psychiatry as a specialty arose from the unique needs of old people with psychiatric disorder and the special knowledge and skills needed to deal with these needs. It differs from general psychiatry not only because of the greatly increased prevalence of dementia in older people but also because the presentation and management of other disorders is different. The pattern of work is also different. Work in interdisciplinary community mental health teams and in partnership with general practitioners, social services, and hospital doctors is a necessary response to the complicated mixture of social, psychological, and medical needs in old people with psychiatric disorder. About three quarters of the referrals to old age psychiatrists come from general practitioners and about a quarter are liaison referrals from hospital departments.

Although old age psychiatry began as a hospital specialty, many old age psychiatrists today are based in the community and give equal emphasis to their community and hospital work. They aim to provide services that are sensitive to the needs of caregivers and patients and also support general practitioners, social services, and other hospital departments. Their work includes the direct assessment and management of disease and the provision of education and information to others working with older adults, aiming to influence the practice of others, as the prevalence of mental illness is far too high for them to deal with it all directly. Three diagnostic groups are responsible for most of the workload: depression, delirium, and dementia.

Depression

Though depression is neither more nor less common in older than younger adults, when it occurs it is more likely to be severe and more likely to need hospital admission. The need for hospital admission probably stems from an interaction of the severity of depression, the higher proportion of old people living alone (about 50% over the age of 75 years), and the frequent coexistence of physical disorder. There is also a higher risk of suicide in old age. Clinically significant depression affects about 10% of old people in the general community, and rates are two or three times higher in selected populations like those in old people's homes or inpatient medical care. About a quarter of the depression seen is quite severe.

The risk of people developing the more severe forms of depression might be reduced by earlier diagnosis and effective treatment in general practice (Box 5.1). Helping general practitioners to be aware of treatable depression in their older patients is a prime educational target for old age psychiatrists (Box 5.2).

The prognosis for untreated depression is relatively poor, so why is some old people's depression undiagnosed and untreated? The evidence currently available suggests that patients and general practitioners concentrate on treatment of physical symptoms. Indeed, depression in older patients commonly presents as a series

---

Box 5.1   Depression in general practice

- The "average" general practitioner with a list size of 1800 and 270 people over the age of 65 will have at least 27 older patients with clinically significant depression, of whom perhaps six will be severely depressed
- Of the 27 older patients who are depressed, six will die over three years and nine will remain persistently or recurrently depressed
- General practitioners are often aware of depression in older patients who come to see them but rarely record this in their notes, prescribe medication, or refer patients with this illness
- Untreated depression in older patients at home has a poor outcome. Mortality is higher than among non-depressed people of the same age, even if the confounding effect of physical illness is allowed for; around a third of depressed older patients are depressed at three year follow up
- Suicide rates are high in old age (especially in men), and old people who attempt suicide more often succeed than their younger counterparts

---

Box 5.2   Elderly people and depression

- Patients presenting with depression with physical symptoms or in association with physical illness respond well to antidepressant drugs
- The more serious side effects and risks can be minimised by prescribing newer antidepressants
- Interactions may be reduced by careful choice of drugs
- Depressed patients in general practice respond well to antidepressants—provided adequate doses are used—and some treatments for physical disorder may be less important than antidepressant treatment

---

of physical problems such as insomnia, tiredness, and repeated minor aches and pains. In addition, depression is commonly associated with physical illness or bereavement and may then be dismissed as "understandable." Doctors are concerned about the side effects and risks of the older antidepressant drugs and possibly the cost of the newer ones, and about polypharmacy and drug interactions. Patients, remembering reports of problems with benzodiazepines, may worry that antidepressants are "addictive." Counselling and psychotherapy services for old people are not generally well developed, and doctors as well as patients may succumb to a feeling of hopelessness and helplessness in the face of social deprivation and multiple diseases.

A first step in improving the management of depression in older adults in general practice would be for each general practitioner to identify depressed patients either opportunistically (they tend to consult more than other patients) or through screening and to record the diagnosis in the notes. Patients who were severely depressed or who remained depressed for more than a few weeks should be considered for treatment with antidepressant drugs and the outcome monitored. Evidence from patients with more severe depression suggests that, in the majority who do respond to antidepressants, there is benefit in continuing treatment for at least two years. The evidence of benefit for continuing treatment of less severe cases is not yet established.

Monitoring, counselling, and, if necessary, antidepressant treatment can also be directed to people who are especially likely to develop depression—for example, those who are socially isolated or recently bereaved or who suffer chronic physical illness. There is a strong link between handicap, associated with disabilities often linked to physical illness and the onset and continuation of depression. For this reason management strategies should aim to reduce handicap and social isolation alongside pharmacological treatment of the depression. Doctors in hospital departments for older people have a special role here, especially with the last group. A number of scales—the geriatric depression scale,[1,2] the brief assessment scale for depression (a card sort scale),[3] and the hospital anxiety depression scale[4,5]— provide a diagnostic indicator and can also be used to measure improvement, though not all are validated as diagnostic instruments in every setting.

In the management of depression, suicide risk should always be ascertained (Fig. 5.1). The patient can be asked, "Have you ever felt so bad that life was not worth living?" and further questions as necessary. If there is doubt about diagnosis, response to treatment, or suicide risk, the opinion of a consultant psychiatrist should be sought. Often the old age psychiatrist will manage depression in the community in partnership with the general practitioner and use support from the community mental health team, psychiatric day hospital for elderly people, and social services.

Where there is risk of suicide, serious self neglect (or, rarely, risk to others), or where the patient is non-compliant or resistant to treatment, hospital admission may be indicated. In hospital a full assessment will include any relevant physical illness, and treatment for those who have not responded to a simple antidepressant regimen may involve lithium augmentation, electroconvulsive therapy, and other treatment. Once a "difficult to treat" depression has resolved, follow up—including adequate continuation therapy,

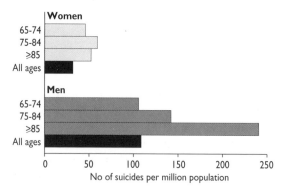

Figure 5.1 Suicide rates are high in old age, especially in men (1993 figures for 10 year age groups over 65 years; source: Office for National Statistics)

monitoring of compliance, and social support—is vital and will be facilitated by the care programme approach.

Delirium

Up to a fifth of older medical inpatients suffer from delirium. It presents as "confusion" or "acute confusional state." It should not be mistaken for dementia and can generally be distinguished by both its acute onset and the presence of acute physical illness. Delirium is particularly common in demented patients, in whom it can be precipitated by relatively minor physical illness and perhaps even by rapid environmental change. Whenever an older patient is seen at home with acute physical illness, delirium should be considered. If it is florid, with disturbed behaviour and hallucinations, it is likely to be noticed. Quieter forms of delirium, with subtle and fluctuating impairment of consciousness and concentration, are more likely to be missed. If they are undetected, especially if the patient lives alone, the delirium may seriously interfere with the effectiveness of treatment for the underlying physical disorder. The doctor may leave the patient at home with a prescription for antibiotics or a diuretic, not realising that the patient will forget to obtain or take the drug.

Delirium may be best managed at home in familiar surroundings, provided that there is adequate social support and the underlying illness does not require hospital services. If admission is necessary, careful management of the transition, with a familiar person accompanying the patient and repeated explanations of what is going on, can minimise the increase in confusion that is common with environmental change.

Dementia

The dementias are common, affecting around 8% of people over 65 years. Prevalence rises rapidly with age, from 2-3% in the 65-69 year age group to over 20% in the over 80s. General practitioners are aware of their patients with the more severe degrees of dementia, but milder dementias are often missed.

The main diagnoses are Alzheimer's disease, vascular dementia, and mixed Alzheimer's disease and vascular dementia. Other patients have a wide variety of disorders, individually rare but important because they are sometimes reversible.

These "reversible dementias" include vitamin B12 and thyroid deficiency, space occupying lesions (including subdural haematoma), normal pressure hydrocephalus, and alcohol related dementia. In addition, a proportion of patients previously diagnosed as having Alzheimer's dementia or vascular dementia have neuropathological changes of diffuse Lewy body dementia. Clinically this group may be distinguished by wide fluctuations in function, extrapyramidal signs and symptoms, and possibly an increased frequency of visual hallucinations. This diagnosis is associated with an abnormal and potentially severe sensitivity to extrapyramidal side effects of neuroleptic drugs.

The exact diagnosis in dementia is of more than academic importance. Vascular dementia is associated with the risk factors for other forms of vascular disorder and may be partly preventable (by controlling hypertension or treating atrial fibrillation with warfarin). When it does occur the development of recurrent cerebral infarction may be slowed down by the use of low dose aspirin. Donepezil is the first drug to be licensed and marketed in the UK for the treatment of dementia. It has a statistically significant but small effect on cognitive function but its place in clinical practice is yet to be established. For this reason, it should probably only be commenced after expert assessment by a psychogeriatrician or neurologist and is best given according to guidelines which include criteria for diagnosis and monitoring of progress as well as an agreement with the patient and relatives about discontinuation of treatment if it is of no benefit to the individual. Potentially reversible dementias, though rare, should be detected and treated as early as possible, before permanent brain damage occurs. Diagnosis is based on history, examination, and investigation.

Diagnosis of dementia

The history includes risk factors (family history, personal history of hypertension or vascular disorder) and the type of onset of the condition (sudden onset suggests delirium or vascular dementia). In regard to the time course of the condition, rapid fluctuation suggests delirium or diffuse Lewy body disorder (and sometimes subdural haematoma); stepwise deterioration suggests vascular dementia; and gradual progress suggests Alzheimer's disease.

To examine for the degree of cognitive impairment, a scale such as the modified abbreviated mental test score (AMT)[6] can be used (Box 5.3). Hypertension, evidence of vascular disease, evidence of stroke, or neurological signs suggest vascular or mixed dementia;

Box 5.3   10 item abbreviated mental test

Ask the patient:

1 Their age
2 The time (to the nearest hour)
3 Address—42 West Street—for recall at end of test: this should be repeated by the patient to ensure that it has been heard correctly
4 Current year
5 Name of hospital (or place the patient is being seen)
6 Recognition of two people
7 Date of birth
8 Years of first world war
9 Name of the present monarch
10 Count backwards from 20 to 1

Scoring: Each correct answer scores one mark. A guide to rating cognitive function: 0–3 severe impairment; 4–7 moderate impairment; 8–10 normal.

---

fluctuation of concentration and level of consciousness suggests delirium or diffuse Lewy body disease. Signs of liver disease may be associated with alcohol use; signs of a mood disorder might indicate depressive "pseudo-dementia." Cortical dysfunction, such as dysphasia, agnosia, or apraxia, suggests Alzheimer's disease or vascular dementia, whereas subcortical dysfunction, such as cognitive slowing or forgetfulness, indicates metabolic or vascular dementia.

Routine investigation consists of metabolic screening, measurement of blood sugar, thyroid function tests, measurement of B12 and folate, and a full blood count. Where indicated, further investigation can include tests of liver function or serological testing for syphilis. Computed tomography can be used when there are atypical features, or to confirm vascular disease or space occupying lesions; but cost and benefits need to be weighed (Box 5.4).

Management of dementia

Once the diagnosis of a number of dementia is made, issues need to be addressed alongside any medical treatment that is appropriate:

- Discussing the diagnosis and prognosis sensitively with patient and caregivers
- Providing information about support services

Box 5.4   The dementias

- Affect 1 in 12 people aged over 65 years
- Prevalence rises with age; more than a fifth of people over 80 are affected
- Severe dementia is rarely overlooked
- Milder dementia may be missed
- Delirium and depression may be misdiagnosed as dementia
- Alzheimer's, vascular, and mixed dementias are commonest
- A variety of other disorders is much less common but sometimes reversible
- Diffuse Lewy body disorder is increasingly diagnosed and important because of neuroleptic sensitivity

---

- Providing information about financial and other legal issues
- Putting the patient and caregivers in touch with services
- Giving the patient and caregivers details of the Alzheimer's Disease Society
- Producing an agreed plan of care, which is revised as often as needed.

Doctors are often shy of discussing the diagnosis with patients, and sensitivity to the patient's wish to know and capacity to understand are central. Caregivers and even patients can be surprisingly relieved to be given the diagnosis of Alzheimer's disease: they may have suspected this for a long time, and it comes as a relief to have the diagnosis. It also enables caregivers to begin to plan for the future. Information is essential for that planning and the Alzheimer's Disease Society produces an excellent set of information and advice sheets that can be copied for patients and carers—every general practice, department of medicine for the elderly, and old age psychiatry service should have both packs. The 20 information sheets cover, among other issues, financial and legal issues; services—who can help; and drugs used for behavioural problems. In the advice series, 19 sheets cover practical topics like communication, wandering, incontinence, aggression, sexual problems, and pressure sores.

Financial matters

Financial matters often cause problems. If the patient is capable of understanding it, an enduring power of attorney may be useful. If the patient is no longer able to understand this and considerable sums of money are involved, the Court of Protection may be the only option.

Difficult behaviour

Wandering, repetition, shouting, inappropriate behaviour, sexual disinhibition, and many other behaviour problems may develop as dementia advances. Each problem needs careful definition. "Wandering," for example, may describe anything from restlessness around the house to a determined commitment to walk to a former abode, even if that means crossing a motorway. An analysis of possible medical reasons for the behaviour should follow: is restlessness due to constipation; is incontinence due to immobility? Behaviour may also only be inappropriate because of impaired understanding—for example, the old man who tries to get into bed with a woman he mistakes for his wife. Depressed mood may produce restless or hostile behaviour. Shouting may be inadvertently reinforced if it brings attention in the otherwise impoverished environment of a nursing or residential home. Behavioural techniques may be useful, but often understanding the meaning of the behaviour for the patient is the clue to devising appropriate management.

Specialist community mental health teams

Specialist community mental health teams for older adults usually include community nurses, psychiatrists, a social worker, and perhaps a psychologist or an occupational therapist. They are well equipped to deal with the more complicated diagnostic and management problems and usually provide a direct link with local day hospital and inpatient services. Most health districts now have specialist consultants in old age psychiatry, though nationally there are about 20 districts without a consultant and many are seriously understaffed for the size of the population covered.

The old age psychiatric service is community focused but acute inpatient beds, day hospital places and some long stay beds still form an integral part of the service and are essential if the community team is to function well. A seamless integration between primary care, community services provided by the community mental health team, social services and inpatient services is the ambition of most psychiatrists in this field. Though it is hard to achieve such a service is good for patients and provides a very satisfying work environment for the team.

37

Under the new community care provisions, social services are expected to make an assessment of the needs of anyone referred to them with mental illness (including dementia) in the community. Increasingly flexible home care services are evolving, though there continue to be funding problems. Local branches of the Alzheimer's Disease Society are a particularly useful source of information and support to carers.

Further reading

Wattis J, Martin C. *Practical psychiatry of old age.* 2nd ed. London: Chapman and Hall, 1993.

Information and advice leaflets are available as a pack (price £4) from the Alzheimer's Disease Society, Gordon House, 10 Green-coat Place, London SW1P 1PH (tel 0171 306 0606).

References

1 Yesavage J, Brink T, Rose T, Lum O, Huang V, Aday M, *et al.* Development and validation of a geriatric depression screening scale: a preliminary report. *J Psychiatr Res* 1983;17:37-49.
2 Herrmann N, Mittmann N, Silver IL, Shulman KI, Busto UA, Shear NH, *et al.* A validation study of the geriatric depression scale short form. *Int J Geriat Psychiatry* 1996;11:457-60.
3 Adshead F, Day Cody D, Pitt B. BASDEC: a novel screening instrument for depression in elderly medical inpatients. *BMJ* 1992;305:397.
4 Kenn C, Wood H, Kucyj M, Wattis JP, Cunane J. Validation of the hospital anxiety and depression rating scale (HADS) in an elderly psychiatric population. *Int J Geriat Psychiatry* 1987;2:189-93.
5 Wattis J, Burn WK, McKenzie FR, Brothwell JA, Davies KN. Correlation between hospital anxiety depression (HAD) scale and other measures of anxiety and depression in geriatric patients. *Int J Geriat Psychiatry* 1994;9:61-3.
6 Hodkinson HM. Evaluation of a mental test score for assessment of mental impairment in the elderly. *Age Ageing* 1972;1:233-8.

6: Rehabilitation and older people

JOHN YOUNG

Rehabilitation is concerned with lessening the impact of disabling conditions. These are particularly common in older people and considerable health gain can be achieved by successful rehabilitation. Hospital doctors and general practitioners should be aware of the core principles of rehabilitation, be able to recognise rehabilitation need in their patients, and have sufficient knowledge of their local rehabilitation services to trigger the referral process.

In Britain, an estimated 4.3 million people over 60 are disabled—this represents 70% of all disabled people and 46% of all older people.[1] Most (over 90%) of older disabled people live in their own homes, and most (over 80%) have only "mild" disability, but many have several types of disability (Fig. 6.1). Disability of all severity grades is strongly related to age, reflecting the increasing prevalence of the common disabling conditions: stroke, arthritis, cardiorespiratory diseases, fractured neck of femur, and peripheral vascular disease.

Rehabilitation is a complex set of processes usually involving several professional disciplines and aimed at improving the quality of life of older people facing daily living difficulties caused by

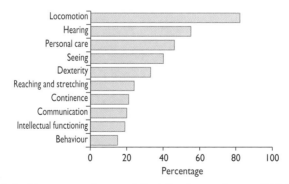

Figure 6.1   Frequency of types of disability in people over 75 living at home

39

chronic disease. The key purposes of rehabilitation can be summarised succinctly:

- Realisation potential
- Re-ablement
- Resettlement
- Role fulfilment
- Readjustment.

Rehabilitation "myths"

The process of rehabilitation is not always well understood. The commonest incorrect assumption is that rehabilitation is time limited, with a clear end point, finishing when the patient leaves hospital. Many patients deteriorate through disease progression, inactivity, new illness, or after a fall, so regular review and reassessment is an important aspect of effective rehabilitation. Another common misunderstanding is that the patient is a passive recipient of a "treatment," as though the therapist were giving them a medicine. Rehabilitation is a highly energetic process in which the patient struggles against his or her disability with guidance from a rehabilitation team. It is not a "quick fix" but requires considerable patience and perseverance. Other myths are that rehabilitation is done only by "therapists" and can be done only in hospital departments; that it is appropriate only for people with mobility problems; that it is too expensive; and that it doesn't work.

Successful rehabilitation

It is easy for the rehabilitation process to focus predominantly on physical functioning. However, successful rehabilitation requires a broader perspective—one which allows social and psychological problems to be identified and addressed (Fig. 6.2).

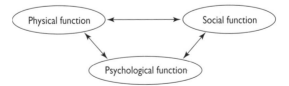

Figure 6.2 Holistic rehabilitation involves more than just physical function

Other success factors for rehabilitation are long established (see also Fig. 6.3):

- A positive attitude and approach
- Individual assessment of patient and caregiver
- Involvement of patient and caregiver
- Team working
- Promotion of independence by:
  Special and general therapeutic techniques
  Optimising the environment

Several easily adopted practical approaches, described below, facilitate these factors and promote more successful rehabilitation outcomes (Fig. 6.4). It is important to realise that rehabilitation involves several overlapping techniques which can be usefully separated into "hard" and "soft." Hard rehabilitation involves some form of "hands on" treatment by a range of rehabilitation staff. Soft rehabilitation is more easily overlooked but is often greatly valued by the patient. It involves talking to, listening to, understanding, and counselling the patient. Some patients require only soft rehabilitation, but a special skill of rehabilitation is to optimise the balance between the two processes.

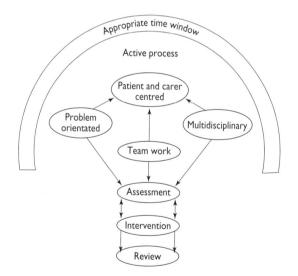

Figure 6.3   Core concepts of rehabilitation

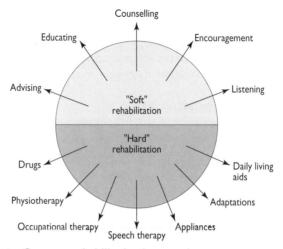

Figure 6.4   Common rehabilitation interventions

Assessment

The classification which has now been widely adopted as a framework to assess patients for rehabilitation is based on four levels: pathology, impairment, disability, and handicap.

Pathology—abnormality of structure or function affecting an organ or organ system—for example, osteoarthritis, ischaemic heart disease.

Impairment—any loss or abnormality of psychological, physiological, or anatomical structure or function—for example, joint pain, breathlessness, muscle weakness, visual impairment, deafness.

Disability—any restriction or lack of ability to perform a task or activity—for example, walking, dressing, going up and down stairs, hearing.

Handicap—the disadvantages for a particular individual resulting from an impairment or disability that limits or prevents fulfilment of a role which is normal for someone of that age, sex or culture—for example, reading a newspaper, going to shops or the pub, gardening, attending a football match, playing the piano.

Doctors tend to be most familiar with uncovering pathologies and impairments ("the diagnosis"), but patients with chronic disease are often more concerned with the consequences of their disease (disability and handicap). Many common aspects of disability can be systematically detected by using the Barthel index

(Box 6.1). Handicap, the particular consequence of the impairments and disabilities to the individual, is best detected by asking open questions such as: "What would you like to be able to do that you cannot do now?" or "What is stopping you going outside?" (fear of falls, too many steps, etc) or "What do you find most frustrating?"

The Barthel index is now widely used in care of older people and rehabilitation departments. It assesses the level of independence or dependence for 10 activities of daily living with a score range of 0 (dependent) to 20 (independent). It is quick and easy to use, has been carefully researched, and aids systematic assessment of disability; when repeated at intervals it can indicate the progress of rehabilitation. The main disadvantages of the Barthel index are that it can be insensitive to change (patients may improve or deteriorate without a change in score) and that it has a low "ceiling" (patients may have a maximum score but still be restricted by inability to go out, cook, clean house, use the bus, etc). Despite these limitations, the Barthel index should be more widely used.

Strengths and weaknesses

Creating opportunities and maintaining a positive attitude is essential in rehabilitation. One simple technique is to consider a disability situation in terms of strengths and weaknesses (Table 6.1). Consider a 77 year old man who has just suffered a hemiplegic stroke and lives with his wife. His strengths and weaknesses can be listed:

When they are set out in this way, it is surprising how often the strengths predominate. They can then be used to address the weaknesses. For example, for this man, occupational therapy input for training in dressing (using the strengths of unsupported sitting balance and wife) and physiotherapy input to teach assisted

Table 6.1

Strengths:	Weaknesses:
Wife as potential caregiver	Unable to stand without help
Can sit unsupported	Unable to walk even with help
Can eat and drink	Unable to dress himself
Continent	Apprehensive about future
Alert	
Previous good health	
Ground floor flat	

Box 6.1   Barthel index

Bowels
0 Incontinent (or needs to be given enema)
1 Occasional accident (once a week)
2 Continent

Bladder
0 Incontinent, or catheterised and unable to manage alone
1 Occasional accident (maximum once per 24 hours)
2 Continent (for more than seven days)

Grooming
0 Needs help with personal care: face, hair, teeth, shaving
1 Independent (implements provided)

Toilet use
0 Dependent
1 Needs some help but can do something alone
2 Independent (on and off, wiping, dressing)

Feeding
0 Unable
1 Needs help in cutting, spreading butter, etc
2 Independent

Transfer
0 Unable—no sitting balance
1 Major help (physical, one or two people); can sit
2 Minor help (verbal or physical)
3 Independent

Mobility
0 Immobile
1 Wheelchair independent, including corners, etc
2 Walks with help (verbal or physical) of one person
3 Independent (but may use an aid)

Dressing
0 Dependent
1 Needs help but can do about half unaided
2 Independent (including buttons, zips, laces, etc)

Stairs
0 Unable
1 Needs help (verbal, physical, carrying aid)
2 Independent up and down

Bathing
0 Dependent
1 Independent (or in shower)

Table 6.2   Goal setting

Who	Mrs Smith	Mrs Brown
Will do what	Walk to her neighbours	Dress herself completely
Under what conditions	Using her Zimmer frame	Without help
To what degree of success	At least once per week	Before 8.30 each morning

transfers (using the strength of the wife as caregiver) would be a positive beginning to the rehabilitation process.

Goal setting

Explicit goal setting is a central task in the management of disabled elderly people. Goal setting should be informed by careful assessment of the patient and precede all rehabilitation interventions (Table 6.2). Successful goals are recognised as being:

- Meaningful—appropriate to the problems and circumstances of the patient
- Agreed—consult and negotiate with patient, caregivers, and rehabilitation team
- Clearly communicated—write them down
- Realistic—challenging but achievable: not everyone can do everything.

A rehabilitation goal is not a vague statement (for example, "we will improve mobility") or a vague action ("we will refer to a physiotherapy department"). A rehabilitation goal is a precise statement and should be constructed so that its achievement is unambiguous.

Barriers to rehabilitation progress

Some patients may not make the amount of progress that was anticipated. Common reasons which should be considered are:

- Unidentified medical problems, such as anaemia, heart failure (fatigue syndrome), undiagnosed Parkinson's disease, undiagnosed hypothyroidism, or the side effects of drugs (especially postural hypotension)
- Occult depression—depression is commonly associated with physical disease in older people but is easily overlooked, and can have important consequences for the patient, who may benefit considerably from treatment with antidepressants (Box 6.2)

- Occult dementia—some patients will have well preserved social skills which mask loss of intellectual function; impairment of memory, concentration, perceptual skills, and apraxia are common in Alzheimer's disease and prevent full cooperation with rehabilitation techniques, many of which are complex learning tasks (see Box 5.3 on p 35)
- Communication problems—check vision (and spectacles); check hearing (and hearing aid).

Remember the caregivers

Caregivers are addressed in Chapter 1. Their contribution needs to be positively acknowledged by purposefully allocating time to understand their perspective and needs. "Knowledge is power"— information giving and contact with support groups are particularly valued. The caregiver may be depressed or anxious and need treatment, and routine discussion of respite care (day or night sitters, rotational care) is recommended.

Box 6.2   Geriatric depression scale

1. Are you basically satisfied with your life?	yes/NO
2. Have you dropped many of your activities and interests?	YES/no
3. Do you feel that your life is empty?	YES/no
4. Do you often get bored?	YES/no
5. Are you in good spirits most of the time?	yes/NO
6. Are you afraid that something bad is going to happen to you?	YES/no
7. Do you feel happy most of the time?	yes/NO
8. Do you often feel helpless?	YES/no
9. Do you prefer to stay at home, rather than going out and doing new things?	YES/no
10. Do you feel you have more problems with memory than most?	YES/no
11. Do you think it is wonderful to be alive now?	yes/NO
12. Do you feel pretty worthless the way you are now?	YES/no
13. Do you feel full of energy?	yes/NO
14. Do you feel that your situation is hopeless?	YES/no
15. Do you think that most people are better off than you are?	YES/no

Scoring: Answers indicating depression are in capitals. Each scores one point. Scores greater than 5 indicate probable depression.

Arranging rehabilitation for older people

The rehabilitation services are characterised nationally by wide variation in availability, type, scope, and content. Several agencies and several departments within these agencies are usually involved, so general practitioners and hospital doctors need to become familiar with their local arrangements. However, selection of patients for referral—and selection of an appropriate rehabilitation service—are practical issues for which guidance in general terms is important.

Selection of patients

Older people with the following should be considered for referral:

- Disability but cause uncertain
- New impairment, disability, or handicap
- Deterioration in existing impairment, disability, or handicap
- Strain on caregiver identified
- Barely coping: residential or nursing home care being considered
- New referral to home care service.

Selection of a rehabilitation service

Many older patients become disabled by an acute illness such as a major stroke, fractured neck of femur, or pneumonia and require emergency hospital admission for medical and rehabilitation care. For other patients, however, it may be less clear whether inpatient or outpatient rehabilitation is most appropriate. Discussion with a general physician or geriatrician, or a prior domiciliary assessment visit, may be helpful in such uncertain circumstances. Key aspects of the decision process are given in Box 6.3.

Outpatient rehabilitation can be organised by referral to an outpatient therapy department, a geriatric day hospital, or a home or community rehabilitation team. In general, clearly defined single problems (difficulty walking, difficulty bathing, etc) can be attended to in outpatient therapy departments but more complex or poorly defined problems, such as "not coping" or falls, are often best managed in a geriatric day hospital. However, care is needed in the referral process as some aspects of impairment and disability are clearly visible (such as knee pain and restricted mobility) but

---

Box 6.3   Considerations for inpatient and outpatient rehabilitation

Inpatient rehabilitation

- High dependency/high care needs (especially night time care)
- Complex or multiple disability
- Rapid response needed
- Poor housing or unsuitable domestic circumstances
- No community rehabilitation available

Outpatient rehabilitation

- Low or modest dependency
- Less complex disability
- Slower response acceptable
- Appropriate housing and domestic circumstances

---

other aspects (such as being unable to do kitchen work) may be hidden. A full disclosure of all important aspects of disability in older people is often best undertaken by a rehabilitation team. This is most usually available via the day hospital.

It has been increasingly recognised that assessment and treatment of older people in their own home has advantages over departmental based assessments. Real daily life problems are more apparent; there is greater opportunity to involve the family; and there is greater opportunity to involve home care and community nursing staff. Some districts now provide separate home rehabilitation teams to achieve this, while in other districts the therapy team is based in the day hospital but much of the assessment and treatment takes place in the patient's home.

Coordination of rehabilitation

Coordination of effort between the members of a multidisciplinary rehabilitation team and between rehabilitation services is important but can be difficult to achieve. It should be easier in hospitals: elderly care wards, rehabilitation wards, stroke, and orthogeriatric units are structures which greatly facilitate team working and coordination between disciplines and agencies. It can be considerably more difficult outside the hospital as natural teams do not usually exist but need to be purposefully formed around individual patients. Consider the common situation of an elderly housebound woman disabled by osteoarthritis who wishes to remain in her terraced council house. A range of services and equipment is required, the access to which may defeat all but the most tenacious of rehabilitation staff. Box 6.4 provides an example.

Rehabilitation research

Although the research base for rehabilitation has expanded considerably, evidence for effectiveness remains patchy. There is evidence to support the general concepts of the rehabilitation process for older people, for stroke units and some evidence to support orthogeriatric units. Several randomised trials of domiciliary rehabilitation have been undertaken with encouragingly positive results.

Perhaps the most surprising finding from the domiciliary rehabilitation studies is how little therapy input is required. Several of the studies used only two or three visits, yet the health gain for the patient was considerable, especially for interventions consisting of occupational therapy (Box 6.5).

Box 6.4   Equipment and services commonly required by older people disabled by osteoarthritis

Equipment/service	*Assessed by/provided by*
● Kitchen aids (tap turner, teapot tipper)	Social service occupational therapist
● Dressing aids (longhandled shoe horn)	Social service occupational therapist
● Pendant alarm	Social service area office
● Frozen meal provision	Home care service
● Walking frame	Physiotherapy service
● Outdoor wheelchair	Wheelchair service
● Ramp to front door	Social service occupational therapist and housing department
● High seat chair	Social service area office
● Raised toilet seat	Social service area office
● Extra stair rail	Social service area office
● Commode	Nursing loans
● Attendance allowance	Department of social services
● Day centre	Social worker
● Day hospital	Consultant geriatrician

Box 6.5   Findings of studies of rehabilitation in the home

Occupational therapy

Bathing aids	Improved independence
Simple aids	Improved independence
Rheumatoid arthritis	Improved independence

Physiotherapy

Falls	Improved balance
Osteoarthritis	Less pain greater mobility
Stroke	Improved mobility and
Parkinson's disease	independence
	Improved mobility

Further reading

Andrews K. *Rehabilitation of older adults.* London: Edward Arnold, 1987.

Squires A, ed. *Rehabilitation of the older patient.* London: Croom Helm, 1988.

Department of Social Security. *Elderly people in the community: their service needs.* London: HMSO, 1985.

Reference

1 Marten J, Meltzer H, Elliot D. The prevalence of disability among adults. London: HMSO, 1989. (OPCS surveys of disability in Great Britain: report 1)

7: Aids to compliance with medication

A J CORLETT

Elderly people may need to take several forms of medication, including tablets and capsules, inhalers, insulin, and eye drops. This chapter describes various aids that are designed to facilitate compliance.

Old people are more likely to suffer from chronic morbidity from multiple diseases. Several diseases may require concurrent drug treatment; polypharmacy is known to be associated with an increased risk of adverse drug reactions, drug interactions, and poor compliance. About 30% of older people are taking three or more medications.

Compliance may be defined as the extent to which a person's behaviour coincides with medical advice. Few patients take their medication as intended by their practitioner; most are partially compliant. Up to 20% of patients do not present their prescription to a pharmacy within one month of issue. Non-compliance is multifactorial and may arise from:

- Not knowing how to take medication (such as orally, twice daily, with food, etc)
- Not understanding the importance of drug treatment in managing disease
- Taking many drugs
- Anticipation or experience of side effects
- Forgetfulness
- Impaired physical function.

Even so, elderly patients with normal cognitive function are more compliant than their younger contemporaries. Simple measures can be taken to improve compliance:

- Educating patients about disease and treatment
- Simplifying drug regimens: minimising the number of drugs and frequency of doses

51

- Using modified or controlled release preparations to decrease dosage frequency
- Involving carers in management of medication
- Telling patients about common early side effects to which they may develop tolerance
- Using drug diaries, calendars, or medication charts
- Using ordinary bottle tops instead of child resistant containers
- Using large print or jumbo labels on containers
- Using compliance aids, such as dose reminders for tablets and devices to help with administration of inhalers, eye drops, etc.

Daily dose reminders and monitored dosage systems

Several types of daily dose reminders are available (see Box 7.1). Most consist of a box divided into days of the week with several compartments for each day—they are suitable for tablets and capsules only. Effervescent, dispersible, buccal, and sublingual preparations or moisture sensitive medicines (such as Omeprazole) cannot be dispensed in compliance devices. Large solid tablets, or multiple tablets taken at a single time, may not fit into the individual compartments. "As required" (PRN) medication, if placed in a daily dose reminder or monitored dosage system, may be taken unnecessarily on a regular basis.

Daily dose reminders are not included in the drug tariff and therefore are not prescribable. Patients or their carers have to purchase the device unless it is dispensed from a hospital.

Some drugs are provided in calendar, "bubble" or "blister" packs. The Medicines Control Agency approves of the dispensing of patient packs—a ready-to-dispense pack with an information leaflet, in accordance with the EC Directive. People with impaired manual function may have difficulty in manipulating the packaging.

The legal and ethical aspects of dispensing medicines into daily dose reminders or monitored dosage systems are not clear.[1] Medicines dispensed directly into daily dose reminders or monitored dosage systems should still comply with current labelling regulations. The labelling should allow identification of each drug in the monitored dosage system, and formulations that look alike should not be dispensed in the monitored dosage system.

Recent data have questioned the stability of medicinal products in compliance devices. Medicines should not be kept in sealed

Box 7.1 Daily dose reminders

Dosett (Ri-med)

- Holds 7 days' medication; marked SUN—SAT (days also marked in Braille)
- Four compartments to each day
- Single daily units are not detachable
- Chart on underside for details of patient's treatment
- Further refinements include a locking device and the Mediset Mini (a pocket sized container with 21 compartments, suitable for small tablets or capsules)
- Though sliding lids on tablet tray have guides, they require considerable dexterity to remove and replace
- Filled weekly by the patient, carer, or pharmacist

Nomad (Surgichem)

- Cassette holds drugs for seven days, with six compartments in each day
- Daily units are not detachable
- Tray is sealed with transparent plastic lid and clear plastic film
- Contains photograph and personal details of patient
- Record of treatment and drug regimen is preprinted on underside of tray
- Filled only under the supervision of a pharmacist

Manrex (Boots)

- Available at Boots and some independent pharmacies
- Medication is heat sealed in large, flat blister packs
- Each pack contains sufficient treatment for 28 days
- Daily units are not detachable
- Packs are colour coded to indicate time of administration—for example, pink indicates morning tablets, white "as required" treatment
- Each pack contains a card with drug dose
- Filled under the supervision of a pharmacist

Monitored dosage systems

53

monitored dosage systems for more than eight weeks. They should be stored in a cool dry place, protected from light, and kept away from children as most of these devices are not child resistant.

Inhalers

Asthma affects about one in 10 older adults. Inhalers are the first line treatment as direct delivery of a drug to the site of action reduces systemic side effects and enables bronchodilating agents to have an immediate action (Fig. 7.1).

Several drug delivery systems are now available.[2] Metered dose inhalers, which are the most widely used, have several disadvantages and may eventually be superseded by breath actuated dry powder systems, which seem to increase the percentage of drug deposition in the lungs. The patient should be instructed in the use of whichever inhaler is prescribed; inhaler technique should be monitored regularly.

Metered dose inhalers

Metered dose inhalers contain up to 200 doses. Discreet and convenient to use, this type of inhaler is preferred by patients. For patients with hand weakness, a lever attachment, Haleraid, may help. Poor inhaler technique is common and has multiple causes. Even with correct technique, up to 80% of the drug is deposited in

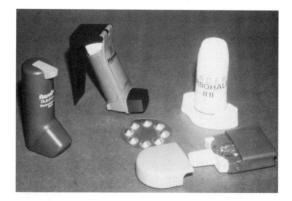

Figure 7.1   Examples of some inhaler devices

the oropharynx; with corticosteroids this may cause oral thrush. Most metered dose inhalers use chlorofluorocarbons (CFCs) as propellants.

Breath actuated metered dose inhalers are similar to standard metered dose inhalers, but more expensive. An automatic spring mechanism is triggered by inspiratory flow rates of 22-36 l/min. Drug delivery is less dependent on inhaler technique.

Spacers are an extension chamber to metered dose inhalers, usually in the form of a plastic bubble. The type of spacer is specific to the type of inhaler. With a spacer there is less drug deposition in the oropharynx and hence a decreased incidence of oral thrush. Spacers increase the proportion of particles inhaled and deposited into the lungs and may be used to deliver larger doses in acute attacks. They may be useful in patients with poor inhalation technique. Larger devices with a oneway valve are most effective but are cumbersome. All devices should be cleaned weekly and replaced every 6–12 months.

Dry powder inhalers

The *Spincap* or *Rotacap* is a small device which breaks open a capsule containing the drug and the lactate carrier. An inspiratory flow rate > 60 l/min is required for effective delivery of the drug, which may be difficult to achieve. Poor technique is common with these inhalers, and they need reloading after each use. The Spincap is less expensive per dose than the equivalent metered dose inhaler; the Rotacap is more expensive.

Diskhalers are larger than metered dose inhalers or dry powder inhalers. A single dose of drug is contained in a blister in an aluminium foil disk; there is a maximum of 8 doses per disk. A dose double that for a metered dose inhaler is usually recommended and an inspiratory flow rate > 60 l/min is required. Diskhalers are expensive and complicated to load.

Turbohalers are small, disposable, breath actuated devices containing up to 200 doses. When only 20 doses remain, there is a warning. For people with arthritic hands, an attachment is available to help turn the base for loading. Turbohalers are simple to use but they are more expensive than metered dose inhalers. Because they deliver pure drug, with no lactate carrier, there is no taste; hence there could be uncertainty that the dose has been taken.

55

Insulin

Six per cent of white people over 65 years (and a much higher proportion of older people from the Indian subcontinent) have diabetes mellitus, and 15–20% are using insulin. Treatment regimens vary from a single morning dose of insulin to four daily doses. The type of insulin used (short, intermediate, long acting, or a combination) and the frequency of administration should be tailored to the needs of the individual patients. Most elderly patients treated with insulin have twice daily injections of a biphasic insulin.

Patients are encouraged to inject themselves, if necessary with supervision from a relative or district nurse, though poor vision may cause difficulty in inserting the needle into the bottle or seeing that the correct amount of insulin has been drawn up. Lack of dexterity in the hands may also cause problems in both drawing up and administering the insulin. Several devices are available to encourage independence.

Magnifiers clip onto the syringe, enlarging the scale and making it easier to see. One device contains two channels: a wider one for the insulin bottle and a smaller one for the syringe—sliding the syringe along the smaller channel guides the needle correctly through the rubber cap and into the bottle. One side of the device shows a magnified image of the scale. Magnifiers are not available on prescription but can be obtained through the diabetic liaison nurse at the local hospital.

Preset glass syringes—Two types of preset syringes are available. These can be set or adjusted by the diabetic liaison or district nurse. They allow the plunger to be drawn back to the set level, so patients with visual impairment can draw up their own insulin. Alternatively the nurse can draw up the dose for the next injection in an ordinary insulin syringe.

Insulin pens are designed to give the patient more flexibility. Various combinations of short and intermediate acting insulin cartridges are available; the pens are either reloaded with new cartridges or are disposable. Reloadable pens are not available on prescription but are available from hospital diabetic clinics.

The maximum quantity of insulin available in a single dose varies from 30 to 78 units, depending on the device. Doses are available in multiples of 1, 2, or 4 units.[3] Accessories to insulin pens are specific to the make of the pen. All patients should have an extra pen as back up and should be able to use an ordinary syringe and insulin phial in case of pen failure. All pens require considerable dexterity.

Examples of a reloadable and a disposable pen are described in Box 7.2.

Eye drops

Glaucoma is the commonest preventable cause of blindness in old age. Unless the patient undergoes surgery, management is by long term use of eye drops. An older person may have difficulty using eye drops because of poor eyesight, arthritis, incoordination, tremor, and fear of the bottle touching the eye. Opticare and Autodrop, shown in Box 7.3, may help in squeezing the bottle or positioning the drop.[4,5] These aids are not available on prescription and have to be purchased; no studies have satisfactorily compared their ease of use and efficacy.

Box 7.2   Insulin pens

B-D pen
- use with Humulin cartridges (5 mixes available in packs of 5 × 1.5 ml cartridges)
- uses B-D microfine needles, available on prescription and from some hospital clinics
- single unit dose up to 30 units
- simple 'dial-press' operation
- easy to read numbers can have magnifier (available from hospital clinics)
- day and night tops available for easy identification of different pens
- spare cartridge provided in carrying case

Penmix 30/70 (5 × 3 ml) pens
- pre-loaded—300 units of insulin (lasts 1 week on average)
- up to 78 units at one time (in multiples of 2 units)
- disposable
- novofine needle

Box 7.3   Help with eye drops

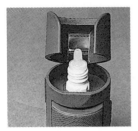

Opticare (Cameron Graham Associates)
- Reusable plastic dispenser fitting most plastic eye drop bottles; fits over the eye and has a finger space for pulling down lower lid
- Squeezing the dispenser requires 25% of the force required to squeeze the bottle
- Difficult to load
- Written instructions provided are poor
- Expensive

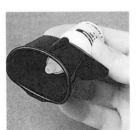

Autodrop (Owen Mumford)
- Clips onto most bottles (except Timolol); holds bottle at correct angle for administering drop
- Lip holds lower lid down; cup fits over eye
- Improves aim by preventing blink reflex during administration
- Easi-drop is similar to Autodrop; it fits onto most bottles (including Timolol) and can be left attached to bottle; an open lattice design allows light to enter the eye during use

References

1 Royal Pharmaceutical Society of Great Britain. *Medicines, ethics and practice; a guide for pharmacists.* London: RPSGB, 1994;12, 9–13, 96.
2 Delivery systems for inhaled drugs in asthma. *Drugs and Therapeutics Bulletin* 1989;27(17):66–8.
3 Pen injections for insulin. *Drugs and Therapeutics Bulletin* 1992;30(1):3–4.
4 Walker R. Aids for eye drop administration. *Pharmaceutical Journal* 1992;249:608.
5 Morrison J. Eye drop aids and counselling sessions for glaucoma patients. *Hospital Pharmacy Practice* 1993;3:413–8.

8: Public transport

T A ROPER, G P MULLEY

Most older people are mobile and able to use public transport without any problems. Those who are hard of hearing or have poor vision and those with mobility problems need not be deterred from using public transport. Though the design and provision of suitable buses, taxis, and trains is not always optimum, many now have imaginative features to help older passengers. Travel by air and sea needs extra planning for disabled elderly people, but helpful advice is available and much can be done to enable even the most disabled traveller to make long journeys confidently and in comfort.

Local travel

Most elderly travellers are able to use all forms of public transport without any problems, but those with impaired mobility and sensory impairments may have some difficulties. A disabled passenger should have the right to unrestricted access to all means of transport and be able to use them with ease and confidence.

Buses

The Disabled Persons Transport Advisory Committee (DPTAC, a statutory body) has consulted disabled people and recommended improvements in the design of buses. These include lower steps; split level steps; "kneeling buses," whose mechanisms can effectively lower the bus and hence decrease step height; better handholds; non-slip floors; and easy to use bell pushes.

Most buses no longer have conductors. Passengers cannot expect physical assistance from drivers, who must stay in their cabs. There are training schemes to make drivers more aware of the needs of disabled travellers—for example, waiting until they are seated before driving off.

Specially adapted buses can take wheelchair users. Assistants help with boarding and securing wheelchairs. Some of these services operate semi-fixed routes and are flexible, allowing travellers to alight near or at their homes. These services also cater for the general public, and fares are charged at standard rates.

In London, the Stationlink service is a circular service that links major rail terminuses in an hourly cycle. The Airbus service links central London with Heathrow Airport and also connects with the Stationlink service. Further information can be obtained from London Transport (whose address is given below).

Senior citizens are eligible for a bus pass and can travel free or at a flat rate. The rate varies from place to place.

Visually impaired travellers may be helped by brightly coloured handrails and good lighting. The Royal National Institute for the Blind (RNIB) has produced signs for hailing buses for their blind members. Some services have produced bus information in Braille and have designed fluorescent bus passes to bring the holder to the instant notice of the driver, who will help by indicating when the destination has been reached. Further information can be obtained from the RNIB.

For hearing impaired and speech impaired people, there are special forms to inform the driver of their destination. These forms are available from local bus operators or local disability organisations.

Taxis

From 1 February 1989 no London taxi could be licensed for the first time unless it could carry a passenger in a wheelchair. From 1 January 2000 all taxis in London are to meet this requirement. The wheelchair rule is statutory in London and can be applied by district councils elsewhere.

Taxis provide door to door service, can be booked in advance, and can be hailed in the street, but they are expensive and not all are accessible to wheelchairs. Taxis that are accessible to wheelchair users have wider door frames and wider angle of opening, and ramps; the rear bench seat tips back to admit the wheelchair user and provide room to manoeuvre more easily; the fixed partition between the driver's and passenger's compartments has been moved forward on the nearside to provide extra space to position the wheelchair; and there are restraints for the wheelchair and a special safety belt for its user.

For blind and partially sighted travellers the RNIB produces signs for hailing taxis.

Community schemes

Dial-a-ride—Most cities have developed a door to door service designed for mobility impaired people that is accessible to wheelchairs. It is for disabled local residents who cannot use public transport. The service has to be booked in advance, and fares are based on local bus rates. The staff are trained to be aware of the needs of disabled people.

Local community transport—Operators have fleets of vehicles which they can hire out to other organisations involved with disabled people to help with outings and excursions.

Shopmobility scheme—Some cities run a shopmobility scheme to maximise disabled shoppers' mobility while in the shopping precinct. Manual or electric wheelchairs and scooters are provided on loan and their use is demonstrated. With sufficient notice an escort can be provided for visually impaired shoppers. Older people who are unable to use a car or public transport may find that shopmobility is integrated with the local dial-a-ride scheme.

Social car scheme—Some authorities run car schemes with volunteers who can drive passengers locally (sometimes further afield). Charges are made on the distance travelled, including the "empty" return journey by the driver.

Voluntary organisations—WRVS (the Women's Royal Voluntary Service), the British Red Cross, St John Ambulance, and Age Concern all have wheelchair accessible transport to transport their members on outings or to hospital. Sometimes they hire out their vehicles.

Distant travel

Elderly people and elderly disabled travellers need to plan ahead to anticipate and minimise potential problems. Before booking a ticket it is worth noting down important questions that need answering to help overcome difficulties that the disabilities might pose. Ask if there are any fare concessions for which they or their escorts may be eligible; ascertain what assistance they can expect at boarding and arrival points; check what facilities are available at the boarding and arrival points—wheelchair accessible toilets, for example.

If the elderly person is going on holiday, determine if the hotel or guest house is suitable and accessible. Holiday insurance is important as medical charges incurred abroad can be expensive; therefore, check that the insurance company specialises in insurance for disabled travellers.

For travel abroad, if continuing medical care is likely to be needed disabled travellers need to check with the travel agents or the British embassy in the country being visited about what medical facilities are available and how to use them.

Rail travel

Check the facilities at both boarding and arrival points: some railway stations may not be staffed or staffed part time or may have spartan facilities for people with impaired mobility. It may be worth travelling further to a mainline station, where the facilities are better and staff are usually available. *Rail Travel for Disabled Passengers* provides information on over 50 principal railway stations and can be obtained from the Disabled Persons Railcard Office or from the Royal Association for Disability and Rehabilitation.

Booking tickets

Make a full declaration of any disabilities when booking tickets. Older people can get concessions if they purchase a senior citizen's railcard, which entitles them to 30% off most standard fares. The current cost is £18. Disabled people can purchase a disabled person's railcard, cost £14. The cost of both cards may increase shortly.

Station facilities

At mainline stations improvements have been made to meet the needs of disabled people. These include the availability of wheelchairs (in London, electric wheelchairs are also available); wheelchair accessible toilets fitted with the national key scheme; level access to catering facilities, with movable seating for the benefit of wheelchair users; handrails on all stairs; car park spaces for disabled travellers, usually near the station entrance; portable ramps to help access to trains. For blind and partially sighted travellers, there are white markings on stair heads and landings, and white lines to mark platform edges. For deaf passengers there are electronic information display systems, induction loops at ticket offices and travel centres, and payphones fitted with induction couplers, which amplify and relay sound to the user's hearing aid, so long as it is fitted with a T switch.

On the train

Intercity trains are nearly all accessible to wheelchairs, with wide access doors and vestibules, grab rails, good lighting, and automatic interior doors. There is usually space for a wheelchair in standard class near the entrance, and opposite this point are seats that can be used for people who need extra leg room. On some lines, trolley services provide refreshments at the passenger's seat.

Some older rolling stock remains in service and is not accessible, so that wheelchair travellers have to travel in the guard's van. There are plans to upgrade these vans to be more comfortable for disabled travellers.

Railway staff cannot help with transfers or getting wheelchairs up and down stairs.

Underground trains

Holders of senior citizen's railcards are entitled to travel free or at reduced rates on the London underground after 9.30 am weekdays and all day Saturday and Sunday. People with a disabled person's railcard and a companion can travel free or at reduced rates at these times.

Some elderly disabled travellers may have difficulties with the automatic gates and may need to use the manual gates. Seats near the doors of a train are clearly identified for elderly and disabled people, and able bodied passengers are requested to give these up if necessary.

Access to some of the deeper lines may be impossible for wheelchair users because of escalators or inadequate lifts. Also wheelchair users are not accepted on the deeper lines because of the potential hazard to them and the other passengers in the event of an emergency, especially if this occurs between stations. On other lines the staff will try to respond to the needs of disabled travellers, especially if they get advance notice. They will also welcome wheelchair users as long as they are accompanied by an able bodied passenger.

Ferry travel

In planning a route it is important to seek advice from motoring organisations. Further advice can be obtained from disabled motoring organisations such as the Disabled Drivers Association, the Disabled Drivers Motoring Club, or the Disabled Motoring Federation.

Disabled people can hire a car to take abroad but they will be charged extra insurance premiums and it may be necessary to take

63

SCHOOL OF MEDICINE & DENTISTRY LIBRARY
ST. BARTHOLOMEW'S HOSPITAL

out special recovery service insurance with the AA or RAC. Cars with hand controls can be hired.

Booking tickets

When booking a ticket a full declaration of any disabilities should be made. Disabled drivers may be eligible for concessions, especially if they are members of associations for disabled drivers; receive the mobility allowance; or own a car with adaptations. A small administration fee may be charged.

Reciprocal parking arrangements exist in western Europe for orange badge holders; they will be able to park with similar advantages as in Britain.

Port facilities

Facilities vary between ports in Britain and on the continent, although these are being slowly improved. Old people need to consider vehicle queueing and parking on the ferry. Other features that have to be considered include whether toilets and public telephones are accessible to wheelchairs.

Facilities on board

More ferries are being equipped with lifts, handrails, and wheelchair accessible facilities, but older ferries may pose difficulties with access, owing to heavy doors, storm sills, narrow gangways, etc. Sealink, North Sea Ferries, Olau Lines, and Sally Lines all have excellent facilities for disabled travellers.

Air travel

The International Air Transport Association (IATA) has over 200 airlines in its membership. Among its responsibilities is a commitment to maintain high levels of air safety. Airlines which are members of the IATA have standardised procedures for acceptance and handling of disabled passengers.

INCAD form

An elderly disabled passenger should inform the relevant airline in advance so it can respond to any special needs. Airlines in IATA have devised a special form called INCAD (incapacitated passengers handling advice) form, which replaces the MEDIF (medical information form). The INCAD form is in two parts: part

1 is completed with information received from the travel agent and gives details of the flight schedule, help required at the airport, help required during boarding and disembarking, and requirements during the flight, such as equipment, oxygen, or a special diet. Usually this information is sufficient but sometimes medical clearance may be required. Part 2 of the form is completed by information supplied by the passenger's general practitioner. A detailed medical account is necessary for the airline's medical adviser, who decides whether an escort is necessary and if clearance to travel will be granted. All information given is confidential.

FREMEC card

Rather than filling in an INCAD form for each journey, a disabled passenger with a chronic stable medical condition who is a frequent traveller may be able to apply for the FREMEC card (frequent traveller's medical card). The card is issued by the medical department of an airline and contains details of the passenger's disability and requirements.

General advice to older air travellers

Before travelling, make a checklist of items required for travel— tickets, passport, travellers' cheques, immunisation certificates, etc. It is also worth listing important items such as the FREMEC card and identity bracelets displaying any illnesses and medication.

It is a wise precaution to avoid alcohol the night before and to avoid flatulent foods, such as beans, 12 hours before the flight. People who require medication should take a plentiful supply for the duration of the holiday, and it should be carried in hand luggage. If continence aids are required, these should also be taken.

It is worth double checking that special arrangements are in place by ringing the airport. Getting to the airport early is advisable.

During the flight it is important for elderly passengers to move their feet to try to prevent deep vein thrombosis. They should make the effort to take short walks down the aisles.

On board

In general, disabled people are boarded first, before able bodied passengers, and are the last to disembark.

Airlines try to accommodate personal preferences and seating requirements. Factors to be considered include ease of transfer from the wheelchair to the seat (some seats have removable arm rests to aid transfers); adequate leg room; and the proximity of the seat to the toilets. Wheelchair dependent travellers may need to be transferred into an aisle chair (a narrow wheelchair) before being wheeled to the toilet.

Flight attendants will try to be helpful, but they cannot assist in toileting, feed patients, or administer drugs or injections.

Disembarking

Usually there is help with baggage and help getting through passport control, either from a travelling escort or from handling staff. If an ambulance is required at the destination, this should be prebooked by the passenger after medical clearance is given by the airline.

Aid for blind and partially sighted passengers

Guide dogs are usually carried free of charge. Most airlines allow them on board to lie by their owner's feet, usually by a window seat. Occasionally an airline will only allow a guide dog to travel in the aircraft hold. Remember that guide dogs are subject to other countries' quarantine laws. Further problems may be caused on return to Britain as the dog will be subject to six months' quarantine.

Aid for hearing impaired passengers

Help with public announcements may be needed, though most information is on television screens now. Passengers wearing hearing aids with a T switch can take advantage of the induction loops fitted at information desks and public telephones.

Contact addresses

Unit for Disabled Passengers, London Transport, 172 Buckingham Palace Road, London SW1W 9TN (tel 0171 918 3312)

Royal National Institute for the Blind, 224 Great Portland Street, London W1N 6AA (tel 0171 388 1266)

National Railcards Office, 3rd Floor, The Podium, 1 Eversholt Street, London NW1 1DN

Royal Association for Disability and Rehabilitation (RADAR),

Unit 12 City Forum, 250 City Road, London EC1V 8AF (tel 0171 250 3222; minicom 0171 250 4119)

Disabled Drivers Association, National Headquarters, Ashwellthorpe, Norwich NR16 1EX (tel 01508 489449)

Disabled Drivers Motoring Club, Cosy Nook, Cottingham Way, Thrapston, Northamptonshire NN14 4PL (tel 01832 734724)

Disabled Motoring Federation, Unit 2a, Atcham Estate, Shrewsbury SY4 4UG (tel 01743 761181)

SCHOOL OF MEDICINE & DENTISTRY LIBRARY
ST. BARTHOLOMEW'S HOSPITAL

9: Money problems and financial help

CHARLIE TEALE

Older people make up the largest low income group in the United Kingdom. This chapter gives an overview of financial help available for older people, including general information, such as pensions and low income benefits, and also particular support for those with disabilities, such as attendance allowance and assistance with residential or nursing home fees. Advice on an individual's entitlements is available from the Benefits Agency and, particularly for those with disabilities, from social workers.

Financial security is one of the keys to being able to enjoy one's later years. Although older people with occupational pensions may be well provided for, those without may face financial hardship. There are over 10 million people of pensionable age in the United Kingdom (currently age 60 for women and 65 for men). Over 1.5 million people aged 60 years and over receive income support because of low income, in addition to which at least half a million who are eligible for this do not claim. This makes older people the largest low income group in the country (Box 9.1). This chapter summarises benefits and financial support available for older

---

Box 9.1   Financial status of older people

- 1 575 000 people aged 60 years and over receive income support (1991)
- Basic state pension is 20% (single) and 32% (couple) of average adult full time wage (1992–3)
- Over half of pensioner households depend on the state pension for at least 75% of their income (1991)
- The Department of Social Security estimates that 33% of pensioners who are entitled to income support and 18% entitled to housing benefit did not claim (1989)
- Pensioners spend more than twice the proportion of their outgoings on fuel, light, and power as non-pensioner households (1991)

people with details on how to find out about allowances and how to get them.

Retirement pensions and widow's benefits

People of pensionable age who have paid sufficient national insurance contributions are eligible for the basic pension; those with lesser contributions may receive a reduced pension. A married woman can claim a pension on her husband's contributions. Divorced people may be entitled to receive a pension, or increase their own pension, on the basis of their former spouse's contributions.

Widow's benefits are based on husband's contributions. A widow's payment of £1000 plus a widow's pension may be payable on the husband's death.

Contributions between 1961 and 1975 and after 1978 may qualify people for graduated or additional pensions, or both. People aged 80 years and over receive an additional 25 pence per week and often qualify for a special non-contributory weekly pension of at least £37.35 (Box 9.2).

Low income benefits

Low income benefits are based on people's incomes and savings but not national insurance contributions.

Income support

Income support is designed to provide a financial "safety net" to bring people up to a minimum weekly income and qualify them for other benefits. National insurance contributions do not have to have been paid in order to qualify. Income support may be paid to people with a low income and less than £8000 (£16 000 for

---

Box 9.2   Weekly payments of full retirement state pensions (Based on 1995-6 rates)

- Basic pension: £62.45
- Basic pension for woman on husband's national insurance: £37.35
- Widow's pension: £62.45
- Additional payment for people 80 years and older: 25p

Box 9.3   Criteria for eligibility for income support

- Savings less than £8000 (£16 000 for permanent residents of care homes)
- Low income
- Working for less than 16 hours a week or not working at all

---

permanent residents of care homes) of savings who work for less than 16 hours a week or do not work at all. Income support is calculated on the basis of age, disability, and savings above £3000; home owners may receive additional payments towards mortgage interest payments or loans for improvements or repairs. Non-disabled people of pensionable age may be eligible for income support if their income is less than £68.80 to £75.70 for a single person, or £106.80 to £115.15 for a couple, depending on their age; these levels may be increased if people are disabled (Box 9.3).

Help with housing and council tax

Council tax benefit can reduce the amount of council tax paid. Housing benefit may help towards rent payments and certain service charges. People eligible for income support are normally entitled to these benefits, and those who do not qualify for income support may receive some help. Eligibility depends on age, income, savings (savings of £3000 to £16 000 will affect benefit; people with savings of more than £16 000 are not eligible), disability, number of people in the family, and levels of rent and council tax. Local councils may also give grants towards home repairs or improvements.

People who live alone may be eligible for a council tax reduction of around 25%. Discounts may be available if the second resident person is a carer or is mentally handicapped (including people with dementia). People who are severely mentally handicapped may be exempt from paying council tax. General practitioners should suggest to the family of patients with moderate or severe dementia that they apply for exemption from council tax.

The social fund

The social fund provides lump sum payments towards specific expenses. Eligibility usually depends on being entitled to income support; savings of more than £1000 are taken into account.

Box 9.4   The social fund provides cash payments towards some expenses

- Cold weather payments: £10 a week on especially cold weeks
- Community care grants: towards cookers, beds, removal, or travel costs to help people live independently at home
- Funeral payments
- Budgeting or crisis loans; help with special item or emergency (must be repaid but are interest free)

People receiving housing benefit or council tax benefit also qualify for funeral payments.

Cold weather payments and funeral payments are mandatory if people meet the requirements. The rest are discretionary (Box 9.4).

Health related costs

Prescriptions are free to people of pensionable age. Those in receipt of income support qualify for free travel costs to hospital (for treatment); free dental treatment, prescriptions, and sight tests; and help towards the cost of glasses. If they are not receiving income support, people with savings of less than £8000 can apply for a certificate of low income entitlement by filling in form AG1 (available from general practitioners, hospitals, dentists, or the benefits agency office). The resulting certificate AG2 entitles the person to the same financial help as someone on income support, while certificate AG3 offers more limited financial support.

Other benefits

Costs such as water rates, fuel, and telephone bills are intended to be covered by income support. There may be additional grants available towards telephone charges, draught proofing, and insulation (to a maximum of about £300).

Benefits for people with disabilities

Attendance allowance

An attendance allowance is payable to people of 65 years and over with a physical or mental disability who need supervision or help with personal care—for example, washing, dressing, or

71

moving around. Although the payment is to the disabled person, the recipients often use it to pay the carer or relative, and increasingly it is being used to buy community services (such as help with bathing). It is payable at two rates: £33.10 for help during the day or night and £49.50 for help both day and night. The conditions must normally have been met for six months, although this is waived for terminally ill people. During this six month period no benefit is paid.

The attendance allowance is not paid retrospectively and is not means tested. It is not taxable and does not depend on national insurance contributions. If people are at home for less than four weeks (as a result of admission to hospital or residential home for respite care) then the whole of the allowance for that period is lost.

Attendance allowance is not a charity but a right. Remember to ask disabled people if they are receiving it. Much resentment occurs if no one tells the family about this entitlement.

Disability living allowance and invalid care allowance

The disability living allowance is an allowance for people disabled before the age of 65 and claimed before they reach 65. It can be available for life or a fixed term. It has two components:

- mobility payments at two levels: £13.15 or £34.60 and
- care payments at three levels: £13.15, £34.60 or £49.50.

The level of payment depends on the degree of disability. The allowance is not available to the biggest group of disabled people, those who become disabled after the age of 65.

The invalid care allowance of £37.35 is usually paid to carers unable to work full time because they care for someone in receipt of the disability living or attendance allowance (at the higher levels); eligibility takes account of other benefits or pensions and is not paid to carers earning more than £50 a week.

Incapacity benefit

Incapacity benefit is for people under state pension age who cannot work because of an illness or disability. It is not payable to those over the state pension age when their illness began but those becoming ill before reaching pension age may receive short term incapacity benefit paid at the retirement pension rate for up to one year of incapacity.

Box 9.5 Summary of benefits for people with disabilities (Based on 1995-6 rates)

- Attendance allowance: £33.10 or £49.50
- Disability living allowance (mobility): £34.60 or £13.15
- Disability living allowance (care): £13.15, £33.10 or £49.50
- Invalid care allowance: £37.35
- Severe disablement allowance: £37.75

Severe disablement allowance—Severely disabled people who have not paid enough contributions may qualify for the severe disablement allowance. This has a basic rate of £37.75 (Box 9.5).

Help with residential or nursing home fees

People wishing to enter a residential or nursing home who require help with the fees are assessed by the local authority which, based on their own criteria, may agree to fund a place. Individual contributions are based on criteria similar to those governing income support. When savings and capital exceed £16 000 the person pays the full fee; when savings fall below £16 000 the local authority will top up the difference after income support—including the residential allowance—has been paid, but it will require a contribution from savings (of £1 a week for every £250 above £10 000) leaving at least £13.75 a week for personal expenses. No contribution is required when savings fall below £10 000.

Until recently an occupational pension was taken into consideration in the financial assessment and used to fund care, leaving none of it for the spouse. New legislation which came into force in 1996 means that only half of the occupational pension need be used towards funding such care. The value of a house is counted in a person's savings unless it is occupied by a spouse or an elderly or incapacitated relative, although this may be waived in certain circumstances. Local authorities have the freedom to pay additional sums towards more flexible care packages (for example, to buy in private care) to allow disabled people to remain in their own homes.

People who lived in a private residential or nursing home before 1 April 1993 have "preserved rights" to higher levels of income support to help pay fees. The level of income support depends on savings, income, and type of home. Income support will top up

---

Box 9.6   Additional financial help

● *Travel*
Train: 1/3 reduction with senior railcard (£18)
Buses: Free or reduced fares are offered by some councils
Coach and plane: Selected reductions

● *Television*
£1.25 reduction in annual licence fee for registered blind people

● *Others*
Selective reductions: cinemas, theatres, museums, leisure facilities, adult education

---

pensions to £208 for residential homes (high dependency rate £240) and £311 for nursing homes (higher rates apply for homes in Greater London). Savings between £10 000 and £16 000 lead to reductions in income support toward residential and nursing home fees; above £16 000 the full fee must be paid.

Further information, leaflets, and claim forms regarding all benefits can be obtained from the local Departments of Social Security or Social Services, or the Citizens Advice Bureau Services Office. Benefit levels quoted refer to the financial year 1997–8.

Further information and reading

Many leaflets and booklets are published by the Department of Social Security and the Benefits Agency; these are available from social security offices.

Age Concern produces helpful leaflets and books on various financial areas, including the book *Know your rights: a guide to money rights for older people* by Sally West; these are available from local Age Concern centres or Age Concern England, 1268 London Road, London SW16 4ER.

10: Care homes

P WANKLYN

Introduction

Long stay care for older people has changed dramatically in the past 25 years. The trend has been for a reduction in the numbers of long stay geriatric medicine beds and local authority residential home places, with an increased provision by the private sector. Private care capacity rose sharply in the 1980s due to open ended income support funding. The community care reforms in 1993 gave local authorities the responsibility for residential care but funds were limited so the growth in private home places was attenuated.

Meeting the costs of long term care will be a challenge for the coming century. The current system of funding is complex and involves local authority and health service budgets. The whole system is to be reviewed and the options include modified means testing in which, for example, all care and health services are free and residential costs means tested, compulsory care insurance, housing equity release schemes, or private long term care insurance.

This article provides an overview of care home provision for older people.

Moving

If an older person is thinking of moving to specialised housing, all the housing options should be discussed with the individual and their carers. Advice is available from a number of sources:

- general practitioners
- the local social services department
- the registration officer for residential homes at the social services department
- the registration officer for nursing homes at the district health authority
- Age Concern, the Community Health Council, Yellow Pages, Citizen's Advice Bureaux, or local voluntary support groups and charities (such as the Alzheimer's Disease Society and the Carers

Inspection and standards

All care homes must be registered and inspected according to the Registered Homes Act, 1984. This act gives general guidance on standards in areas such as accommodation, fire and accident prevention, and/or, safety, and staffing. Health authorities are responsible for the registration and inspection of local nursing homes. Local authorities have set up semi-autonomous units to register and inspect all residential homes within their area. Responsibility for detailed interpretation of the standards is devolved to the local inspection units. The Burgner Review, 1996, made a number of recommendations including the setting of more explicit national benchmarks for standards in residential homes, and developing a common framework for regulating residential and nursing homes.

Registration

The registration procedure establishes whether the applicant is a 'fit person' and that the home and its operating policy will meet the local standards. Once these requirements are satisfied, a registration certificate is issued which will stipulate the maximum number of places in the home for residents with certain levels of need.

The person in charge of running a nursing home may not be the registered person but must always be a registered medical practitioner or qualified nurse.

Inspection

Each home receives two inspection visits per year, one of which is unannounced. At present, reports of individual residential homes but not nursing homes are available to the public. Lay individuals are now involved with the inspection of residential homes but not nursing homes.

The British Geriatrics Society[2] has stated that homes should provide:

- personal choice in food, clothing, forms of address, social activities, daily routine, general practitioner
- privacy
- an easily accessible complaints procedure
- an advocacy system for residents
- personal control of finance and medication where possible
- access to a full range of diversional activities

- access to community, health, and social services
- an individualised care plan.

Some inspection units are now assessing how individual homes are fulfilling these objectives.

Finance

Anyone may approach a care home directly if they are able to make the arrangements and pay the fees. However, if their capital falls below £16 000, local authority support should be sought. There may be problems obtaining this support particularly if the cost of the home exceeds the local 'standard' rate and there is no other source of additional funding. For this reason the local authority should be contacted in advance if there is any chance of funding running out.

A person with capital totalling more than £16 000 pays the full fees; when capital falls between £10 000 and £16 000 the local authority will pay part of the fees. Capital less than £10 000 is ignored but a contribution from income (including benefits) will still be required. A personal expenses allowance of £13.10 per week should remain.

If the local authority agrees for a person to enter a care home, it will usually suggest a choice of suitable homes. However, if the person has chosen a different home the local authority must arrange a place there if it is suitable for the person needs, and does not cost more than the local authority would normally pay. If the preferred accommodation does cost more, a place may still be arranged if a third party is able to make up the difference in cost.

Housing for people with special needs

Older mentally infirm people

Some homes cater for people with dementia or are registered also to take people with physical disabilities. Nursing staff should have suitable training in mental illness.

Visual impairment

The Royal National Institute for the Blind and other societies for the blind have worked with housing providers to develop sheltered schemes for people with visual impairment; they also provide four residential homes. The Royal National Institute for the Blind will supply a list of suitable residential and holiday accommodation for blind people.

People who use wheelchairs

People who use wheelchairs require well designed housing with good access via ramps to wide doorways, and adequate circulation space in hallways. Modifications may be needed to the bathroom, and sockets, switches, and surfaces should be at waist height. The statutory building regulations relating to accessibility and adaptability of new buildings and housing is an issue which is currently being reviewed.

Ethnic minority needs

Few housing associations or homes cater for specific social, cultural, dietary, and religious needs of ethnic minorities. The Housing Corporation provides a list of registered housing associations which cater for people from ethnic minorities.

Age Concern produces a series of numbered factsheets related to care homes:

Local authority charging procedures for residential and nursing home care, factsheet number 10

Financial support for people in residential and nursing homes prior to 1 April 1993, factsheet number 11

Finding residential and nursing home accommodation, factsheet number 29

References

1 Davies K. Emergency alarms. In: Mulley G, ed. *More everyday aids and appliances.* London: BMJ Publications, 1991:39–45.
2 British Geriatrics Society. Policy statement number 4: private and voluntary homes. London: British Geriatrics Society, 1990.

11: Housing for older people

P WANKLYN

Introduction

Standards of housing may affect not only quality of life, but also the survival of elderly people.[1] A recent housing survey found that 10% of people aged over 65 were living in the worst housing category and although this is the same proportion as the general population, it still represents around 700 000 households.[2] In this country most older people live independently in either private or rented accommodation, but the rate of institutionalisation rises sharply over the age of 85 (Table 11.1).[3]

As the proportion of the 'oldest old' rises, the provision of appropriate housing will become increasingly important. Health professionals should be aware of the range of housing options open to older people; these will be discussed in this article.

Older people's views on housing

Qualitative research and surveys have highlighted those factors which influence older people's satisfaction with housing:[4]

- renting or owning a house is less important than its quality and environs
- damp and cold are particular sources of dissatisfaction and improvements to heating and insulation are considered a priority

Table 11.1 Institutional care in long stay hospital bed or residential and, or, nursing home, Great Britain, 1991[3]

Age (years)	Percentage of people in institutional care		
	Male	Female	Combined
65–79	1.1	1.0	1.0
70–74	1.6	1.9	1.8
75–79	3.0	4.4	3.8
80–84	6.2	10.3	8.9
85 +	15.2	26.3	23.7
All 65 +	3.0	6.4	5.0

- the size of a house is less important than its type—for example, bungalows are more popular than ground floor flats, the latter being the least popular type of accommodation
- a toilet on the same level as the living space is important and a bathroom with a bath and a free-standing shower or separate shower room are desirable
- kitchen layout that minimises the need to bend and stretch—for example, to cupboards
- close neighbours
- the presence of good local shops and public transport

Housing design

Functional decline in activities of daily living frequently necessitates adaptations to the home if continued independence is to be possible. At present, very few building companies include design features in new homes which would enable them to be easily adapted for a disabled person.[5] Such features might include:

- wheelchair accessibility taking into account such factors as distance from the road, the gradient, and the door width
- plumbing for downstairs shower and/or, toilet
- suitably positioned switches, power points, heating controls, and meters for wheelchair users
- changes to wall design allowing for fixing rails or a stair lift.

People with visual impairment need particular consideration with regard to housing design, and advice is available from the Royal National Institute for the Blind Housing Service. Special adaptations to a home for a visually impaired person should include:

- recommended light levels without large variations; glare may be reduced by the careful positioning of light sources, the use of a non-reflective wall and floor finish
- use of colour/tone contrast to help in identifying objects such as signs, work surfaces, switches, and doors
- adequate lighting for stairs, with lights positioned to give contrast between the treads and the risers; also colour/tone contrasted nosing to step and hand rails
- inclusion of door closers, rounded edges, and passages with no obstructions
- no unguarded projections above waist height.

Repairs and adaptations

Home repairs may be overlooked by some older people because of poverty or disability, and housing grants are given least frequently to people aged over 75. Older home owners can get advice about repairs or adaptations from several sources:

- housing agency services, sometimes called 'Care and repair' or 'Staying put', give practical advice to older home owners on arranging surveys and grant applications, obtaining estimates, and monitoring work as it proceeds. Although these agencies are non-profit making, a charge may be made; this charge can be included in a grant or loan application
- Citizen's Advice Bureaux
- The housing or environmental health department of the local council for information on ways to get help with paying for repairs and improvements

If adaptations are needed to a home because of disability, the local social services department will arrange an assessment by a community occupational therapist.

Grants

To help pay for repairs or adaptations to a home, there are three main housing grants available from the local authority: a house renovation grant, a home repair assistance grant, and a disabled facilities grant. Application for these grants is through the housing or environmental health department, and two written competitive quotes should be obtained for the work. It is important not to allow any work to start until the grant has been approved.

House renovation grant

A house renovation grant is means tested and discretionary. The grant is available to owner occupiers, certain tenants, and landlords, and may be used to make a building fit for habitation, or for certain essential replacements—for example, wiring, guttering, damp proof course, and repairs to structure such as the roof, walls, foundations, or stairs. A house renovation grant can also be used for heating, insulation (if the house is in good repair, a house repair assistance grant or home energy efficiency scheme grant would be more appropriate) or work on inconvenient features such as a steep staircase or low doorway.

83

Home repair assistance grant

A home repair assistance grant is discretionary and limited to £2000 per application and £4000 per property over three years. The grant is given for repairs or adaptations to a home occupied by a person aged over 60, or to younger people who are disabled or receiving benefit. There are many potential uses for the home repair assistance grant including weatherproofing, insulation, crime prevention measures, door and/or, window repair, and provision of wheelchair ramps and rails.

Disabled facilities grant

A disabled facilities grant is available to people who have been assessed as having a disability, not necessarily registered disabled, and are means tested. The grant is mandatory if the disabled

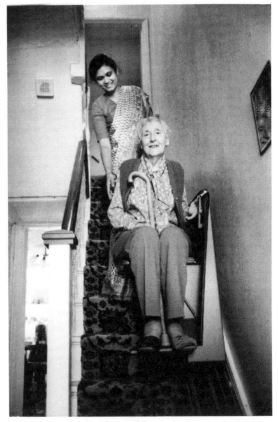

Figure 11.1 Adaptations, such as lifts and alarm systems, may allow people to stay in their own homes. Reproduced courtesy of Ulrike Preuss.

and are means tested. The grant is mandatory if the disabled person does not have full access to the property and its amenities. It can be used to provide easier access to and wit hin the home, kitchen and bathroom facilities for independent use, and for improving and adapting heating and lighting. The grant is discretionary for a wider range of work and ensures that the home is suitable as accommodation, for employment, and for welfare needs.

If there are problems in obtaining any of these grants, contact the local social services department or the Royal Association for Disability and Rehabilitation.

Security

Older people are less likely to be the victims of burglary or violent crimes yet are most concerned about crime and security. Every police station has a Crime Prevention Officer who can visit the home to give general advice and provide information on securing doors and windows with suitable locks, and installing extra lighting and burglar alarms. Some local councils and voluntary organisations also produce leaflets on security measures, and may even give grants to help make a house more secure. There are no specific grants available for security measures on a national basis but a home repair assistance grant may be provided by the local authority.

Heating

The home energy efficiency scheme

The home energy efficiency scheme provides grants for insulation including changing loft insulation from 50 mm to 150 mm, and draughtproofing up to a current maximum of £315. This grant is available to all people who are receiving benefits. People who are aged over 60 but not receiving benefits are eligible for a lower grant of up to £78.75. Further advice about the grant and local approved 'network installers' is available from the Energy Action Grants Agency.

The Social Fund

The Social Fund provides loans and grants mainly to people receiving income support; some of the funds may be used for certain heating systems or fuel bills. To meet the cost of extra fuel during cold spells, payments of £8.50 per week of cold weather are also made to people aged over 60 receiving income support.

Further advice on financial help with heating costs and ways of keeping warm are given in Age Concern's factsheet number 1. The Winter Warmthline (freephone 0800 289404) provides information on heating between October and March.

Specialised housing

The legal rights of people who rent accommodation are important to consider, as feeling secure is crucial for many older people (Age Concern factsheet number 35). There are two sorts of agreement; tenancies and licenses.

Council and housing association tenants

People who rent council or housing association accommodation are usually tenants. Almost all council tenants, and housing association tenants who moved in before 1989, have secure tenancies. The grounds for the landlord to seek repossession are mainly discretionary. Those people who became housing association tenants after 1989 usually have assured periodic tenancies. There is no fixed length for the tenancy and less protection against unreasonable rent increases.

Licensees

Licensees have fewer rights than tenants as the housing agreement simply implies permission to stay in a property. However, the landlord must give notice of the intention to regain possession of the property but does not need a court order to do so; court orders are required for tenants.

If a person is asked to leave their home, it is essential that they seek advice.

Sheltered housing

Sheltered housing is available to rent or buy, but it is usually in short supply.

Sheltered housing developments provide varied levels of care and support from specifically designed housing with no communal facilities to units with wardens and extra care facilities such as meals, home care, or visits from the district nurse.

Many sheltered housing developments were built by local authorities in the 1960s and 1970s but housing associations now run 31% of the total stock. Housing associations have tended to produce smaller dwellings comprising fewer bungalows but more flats than the local authorities.

The housing corporation is the national organisation regulating housing associations. It also works with housing departments to ensure that appropriate housing is developed, and funds research projects related to housing issues. Sheltered housing developments usually consist of self-contained flats, bungalows, or houses in developments of 24 to 40 properties. An average sheltered housing scheme consists of 25% bedsitters, 66% one-bedroomed dwellings, and 8% two-bedroomed dwellings.[6] Sheltered housing is purpose built for older people so features may include flat or ramped access, sockets and switches at waist height, walk-in showers, and grab rails. The housing development may also include a guest room, common room, and laundry, as well as a resident warden (see Box 11.1) and alarm system, but meals are not normally provided. Pets are sometimes allowed. For tenants, a service charge is payable to the landlord for the warden, alarm system, and maintenance and cleaning of communal areas and grounds. Leaseholders also pay a similar service charge to the management organisation which may also include a 'sinking fund' to cover the costs of long term maintenance.

Abbeyfield Society

The Abbeyfield Society is a national organisation comprising 600 local societies run by volunteers. The society provides sheltered housing in a 'supportive' environment, and also residential care homes. Abbeyfield houses tend to be large and accommodate eight to 12 residents who eat communally the main meals prepared by a resident housekeeper. There is no 24-hour staff cover or personal care except for short term assistance or emergencies. The weekly charge tends to be higher than other

---

Box 11.1   Functions of a warden in sheltered housing

- visits daily
- no obligation to provide personal assistance
- not a proxy relative
- will contact relatives and/or, general practitioner if problems occur

---

sheltered housing. Residents have traditionally been licensees but there is a move to providing tenancy agreements. It is wise to obtain advice from a solicitor, Citizens' Advice Bureaux or housing advice centre if considering applying for residency in an Abbeyfield house.

Almshouses

Most almshouses have been in existence for centuries, and many consider only particular applicants, depending on conditions given by the original benefactor. Accommodation is provided rent free but a weekly contribution for upkeep may be required.

Trustees manage a group of almshouses, and standards vary considerably between groups. Residents are legally considered to be licensees so again tenure is less secure than with a housing association.

Further reading

The following publications are available from Age Concern England, Astral House, 1268 London Road, London SW16 4ER
Bookbinder D. *Housing options for older people, 1991.*
A buyer's guide to sheltered housing, 1995
Help with heating, factsheet number 1
Retirement housing for sale, factsheet number 2
Rented accommodation for older people, factsheet number 8
Older home owners: financial help with repairs and adaptations, factsheet number 13
Feeling safer at home and outside, factsheet number 33
Rights for council and housing association tenants, factsheet number 35

Useful addresses

Care and Repair England, Castle House, Kirtley Drive, Nottingham NG7 1LD (tel 0115 9799091).
Energy Action Grants Agency, Freepost, PO Box 130, Newcastle upon Tyne NE99 2RP (tel 0800 0720150).
Abbeyfield Society, Abbeyfield House, 53 Victoria St, St Albans, Hertfordshire AL1 3UW (tel 01727 857536).
Almshouse Association, Billingbear Lodge, Carter's Hill, Wokingham, Berkshire RG40 5RU (tel 01344 452922).
Housing Corporation, Head Office, 149 Tottenham Court Road,

London W1P 0BN (tel 0171 3932000).
RNIB Housing Service, Garrow House, 190 Kensal Road, London
W10 5BT (tel 0181 9692380).
Elderly Accommodation Counsel, 46a Chiswick High Road,
London W4 1SZ (tel 0181 7421182).

References

1 Zhao L, Tatara K, Kuroda K, Takayama Y. Mortality of frail elderly people living at home in relation to housing conditions. *J Epidemiol Community Health* 1993;47:298–302.
2 Department of the Environment. *English house condition survey 1991*. London: HMSO, 1993.
3 OPCS, 1991 Census; Communal Establishments, Great Britain, 1993.
4 Wilson D, Aspinall P, Murie A. *Factors influencing housing satisfaction among older people*. University of Birmingham: Centre for Urban and Regional Studies, 1995.
5 Frain J, Carr P. Is the typical modern house designed for disabled older people? *Age Ageing* 1996;25:398–401.
6 Elderly Accommodation Counsel. *Sheltered housing in England: An overview of provision, 1994*.

12: Carers

ANNE F TRAVERS

Caring by families and friends is the backbone of community care. Carers face physical, emotional, social, and financial problems. They need recognition, information, and support from the health professionals with whom they and the person they care for come in contact. Much information is available to assist carers and to enable their doctors to help them in their caring role.

> "The primary sources of support and care for elderly people are informal and voluntary. These spring from the personal ties of kinship, friendship and neighbourhood . . . . Care in the community must increasingly mean care by the community."
>
> *Growing Older*, 1981[1]

Since the 1950s there has been a gradual shift in the provision of care from hospitals to care in the community. A large proportion of community care is "informal," provided mainly by family. The general household surveys of 1985 and 1990 showed that there are as many as six million carers in Great Britain, providing varying degrees of care. The transition to the caring role is often slow, following the older person's physiological decline and gradual accumulation of diseases. However, some people are precipitated into caring for an older person—for example, when that person suffers a stroke.

Who cares?

Caring is an activity spanning all age groups. There is increasing concern over (and action for) young carers. The peak age for caring is the fifth to seventh decades, but many older people are carers. Over a third of informal care to people over 65 is provided by people over 70. One third of older people can expect to become carers during retirement; they are more likely to provide intimate care and heavy nursing tasks and to care for a spouse.

Both men and women care, although men are considerably less

likely to become carers. Once they have become carers, men and women have similar experiences of caring. If caring is defined as an activity that occupies 20 or more hours per week (to distinguish it from the provision of purely practical help), the prevalence of caring by men rises steadily throughout life, reaching 5-6% by their late 70s, whereas for women it peaks at 7% in their early 60s. The prevalence of caring in ethnic minority communities is not known. It is likely to increase as the number of older people grows during the next decade. Caring spans all social classes, but those with more financial resources and greater skills as advocates for themselves and those they care for are likely to fare better. There is not usually much help to the main or primary carer from other family members or from "the community." Where care is shared, it is rarely shared equally.

There is a spectrum of caring from the heavily involved carers (often older carers and women, providing intensive help to spouses and parents or parents in law) to those carers who provide fewer hours of practical (not personal or physical) assistance to someone living in another household. Most carers of older people belong to the latter category, but about 75% of the total time devoted to informal care comes from carers living in the same household.

Types of care provided

Many carers who provide practical assistance rather than more intimate care are trying to combine their caring responsibilities with paid employment. Their caring work involves activities such as "keeping an eye on" the older person, companionship, shopping, transport, taking out for visits, help with paperwork and finances, and doing repairs and gardening. This group of carers is most unlikely to receive any statutory help.

In contrast, a minority of carers perform intimate personal tasks such as washing, dressing, toileting, and feeding and physical tasks such as lifting and transferring from bed to chair. Training, equipment, and professional advice are usually lacking.

Strains on carers

Older people who need personal and physical care may experience multiple disabilities and problems. In parallel with this, carers face physical, emotional, social, and financial problems. They are more likely than non-carers to have a longstanding illness or disability. The phenomenon of the emotional costs of caring is well documented. Surveys have found as many as half of those carers surveyed to have general health questionnaire scores in the morbid range.[2] Sleep disturbance and difficult behaviour are the two problems independently associated with the greatest degree of strain on the carer. Incontinence, especially faecal incontinence, and many other factors are associated with emotional distress in carers. The stressful effects of sleep disturbance have not been recognised in any policy for substantial provision of night respite or night sitting services.

The social life of those carers providing intensive help is often restricted, partly due to the burden of extra time-consuming work

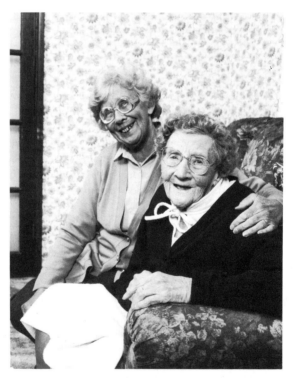

Figure 12.1 Many carers provide practical assistance such as help with shopping or paperwork, transport—or companionship. Reproduced courtesy of Carers National Association.

and partly due to fear of leaving the dependent relative alone or with others. Many carers have not had a holiday for over five years. Particular problems are experienced by carers of people with mental illness, who may feel embarrassed to take the person they care for to a public place.

A Gallup survey of carers drawn from the general population in February 1996 showed that 45% received no help whatsoever with their caring role; 14% received help from social services and 34% from another relative.[3] Carers National Association surveys of known carers in 1994 and 1995 showed that only a quarter had received an assessment in their own right and 60% did not know that they were able to seek their own assessment. Carers were less satisfied with the thoroughness and clarity of explanation of their own assessments than with the assessments of the person cared for. Only 32% of the former and 37% of the latter were confirmed in writing. Only about 40% of the carers considered that the assessment met their own needs.[4]

Finances

In general, carers have poor financial status. An advanced economics of caring has yet to be developed, because conventional economics has ignored all aspects of the informal sector. In 1993, the Institute of Actuaries estimated the value of unpaid care at £33.9 billion a year (compared to £7bn for all institutional care and £3.1bn for professional home care). Carers are often unaware of their entitlements, and the disabled older people for whom they care often are not receiving attendance allowance. Only 250 000 carers receive invalid care allowance. Age has important implications for people's economic resources, so older carers looking after elderly dependants are particularly disadvantaged. The February 1996 Gallup survey showed that, although 63% of those who are not currently carers would expect family or friends to look after them should they become ill or disabled, only 3% thought that their families should be responsible for funding this care. Sixty two per cent thought that the state should pay for the provision of such care and a further 28% that the costs should be shared evenly between family and state.[3]

There is a considerable opportunity cost engendered by the constraints on employment of those caring for older people. Many have difficulties in combining caring with traditional working patterns. In 1993 the Department of Health issued a booklet on employers and carers, emphasising the need for employers to make their management and personnel practices more carer friendly.[5] A further financial problem is the extra expenditure on the older person, which may well exceed the attendance allowance—costs are incurred from extra heating, laundry, and buying in services. Also, the activity of caring itself is associated with an enormous opportunity cost in the time spent caring.

The Carers (Recognition and Services) Act 1995, originally introduced as a private member's bill, came into force on 1 April 1996. The act amends the National Health Service and Community Care Act 1990 in order to create a new duty on local authorities to assess the needs of individual carers (those providing a substantial amount of care on a regular basis) and to enable (but not oblige) the authority to provide appropriate services for carers. No new money has been provided to accompany the new duties. The bill also amends the law to embrace young carers and people caring for disabled children.

What do carers need from the doctor?

Carers need three things—recognition, information, and support—from their general practitioners and from the hospital doctors with whom they and the person they care for come in contact. Support includes respite—necessary breaks from caring.

Many carers do not recognise themselves as such. Many more are not recognised by the health professionals with whom they come into contact. They may be seen just as the "next of kin," and the considerable part they play in the care of the older person is simply not realised.

> "For too long, carers have been the unrecognised partners in our welfare system. Their services have been taken for granted. They have been regarded as a resource but not as people with their own needs. With the greater dependence to be placed by the Government upon care in the community it is time to bring the carers into the mainstream and give them the recognition they deserve. That recognition will inevitably cost money but it is long overdue."
>
> House of Commons Social Services
> Committee, 1990[6]

Carers appreciate acknowledgement of the role they are playing, even a simple listening ear: "How are things going for you, Mrs Brown?" It is worth remembering that carers may not have the same general practitioner as the person for whom they are caring. Carers usually know the person they care for very well. When they sense the beginnings of a new clinical problem for the older person, they appreciate acknowledgement of their concerns and the chance to participate in decision making that does not override the views of the older person.

Carers appreciate honest and up to date information about the diagnosis and prognosis of the person they are looking after, even if the nature of the older person's diseases and disabilities means that the information is incomplete. The provision of such information is also part of the necessary process of working towards the eventual cessation of caring, brought about either by the death of the older person or by his or her entry into permanent residential or nursing care (or, more rarely, by recovery from illness). Giving such information is not intended to break the confidentiality of the doctor-patient relationship and should not ignore the wishes of the older person. Carers also benefit from information about dealing with the everyday physical, behavioural, and emotional problems of caring.

Just as importantly, carers (and the person cared for) need information about the statutory, voluntary, and private provision of services and about the financial benefits available. Doctors and other health professionals cannot be expected to know all the information that every carer needs. However, they should know where the boundaries of their knowledge lie and where to refer the carer for further information and help. Several measures that can be taken to inform carers are listed below.

Advocacy

Some doctors are frightened, unjustifiably, of opening the floodgates if they identify every carer of an older person and refer her or him on to the statutory and voluntary sectors for services and for respite. However, carers can benefit from the advocacy of medical professionals in helping both them and the people they care for to gain access to much-needed services. This is particularly the case for the most disadvantaged carers, who are often elderly themselves: to hold back from referring disabled people and their carers may help to perpetuate the inverse care law (Box 12.1).

Box 12.1   Suggestions for action by medical practitioners

Action in primary care
- Carry out an audit of carer recognition and identification (a pack suitable for general practice is available free from Leeds Carers Health Project, Brunswick Court, Bridge Street, Leeds LS2 7RJ)
- Use a team approach in primary care (the North Yorkshire Health Authority's pack, "Working with Carers" (see information sources) is designed for just this purpose)
- Get a stock of Carers Emergency Cards from the Carers National Association (see below)
- Dedicate a noticeboard to carers' issues:
  Include the contact phone numbers for local and national Carers National Association, Alzheimer's Disease Society, and local carers support groups
  Put information about attendance allowance, invalid care allowance, and disability living allowance on the board
  Put the address and phone number of the local carers' centre (if applicable)
  Highlight both the regional and national carers' weeks
- Start a carers support group based at the practice

Action in both primary and secondary care—wards and clinics
- Ask patients about their hidden roles as carers or cared for. (Do not presume that weekly home care is the mainstay of a patient's "care in the community" nor that the daughter who accompanies her father to see the doctor is a concerned but otherwise inactive relative)
- Get a stock of information packs about local services that your social services department or Carers National Association have produced, and distribute these to the carers you identify —don't wait for them to ask
- Make a small library of the books mentioned here—to provide yourself with answers to the questions that carers raise over the management of such problems as difficult behaviour, repetition, wandering, aggression, and to lend to carers
- Make special arrangements for carers coming for an appointment about their own needs, if the older person cannot be left at home for long

Information sources

Practical information for professionals

- *Working with carers—a resource pack for general practice* (published by North Yorkshire FHSA, 1994). This is a mine of information on what each member of the primary care team can do to support carers. Available from NorthYorkshire Health Authority, 3rd Floor, Ryedale House, 60 Piccadilly, York YO1 1PE (tel 01904 631345); price £5.

- *Age Concern Fact Sheets.* This compilation of 34 information sheets covers an extensive range of practical problems of older people, such as attendance allowance, disability living allowance and housing benefit, help with incontinence, help with heating, sheltered housing for sale, holidays for older people, finding help at home, issues around nursing and residential homes, legal arrangements for managing financial affairs. It is continually updated. Available from Age Concern England, Astral House, 1268 London Road, London SW16 4ER (tel 0181 679 8000); initial subscription for a complete set costs £40.

- *Age Concern Information Circulars.* Monthly bulletins compiling news and information relevant to older people, their carers, and health and social service professionals. Information is grouped under headings such as community care, death and bereavement, disability, health and health services, housing, income, legal affairs, residential, nursing home and long term care, social security. Available from Age Concern England; annual subscription is £19.

Information for carers

- *The Carer's Companion* (written by Richard Corney; published by Winslow, 1994). Written by a clinical psychologist, this book gives excellent advice on dealing with the everyday emotional and practical problems of caring for people with depression, stroke, or dementia. There are comprehensive sections on sexual problems and shorter, helpful sections on toileting difficulties, insomnia, facing hurt and aggression, clinging, and wandering and forgetfulness. Available from Winslow Press, Telford Road, Bicester OX6 0TS; price £7.99.

- *Caring for Someone at Home* (written by Gail Elkington and Jill Harrison; published by Hodder and Stoughton, 1996). Chapters include deciding to care, respite, community care, benefits, financial matters and council tax, health rights, and practical caring difficulties. Available from the Carers National Association (address below); cost £5.99 or £3 to carers when they join the Carers National Association.

- *Caring in a Crisis* is a series of seven handbooks published by Age Concern. The books cover caring for someone who has dementia, who has had a stroke, who is dying, who is going home from hospital, choices for the carer, what to do and who to turn to, and finding and paying for residential and nursing home care. Available from Age Concern's mail order unit (address above); each book costs £5.95 or £6.95; the complete set costs £39.95.

- *Pensioners and Carers* (written by Paul Brown, Anne Mountfield, and Alka Patel; published by the Directory of Social Change, London, 1995). This book, which is addressed to the older person rather than the carer, includes comprehensive accounts of state benefits and grant making charities. Available from DSC Books, 24 Stephenson Way, London NW1 2DP (tel 0171 209 5151); price £15.95.

- *Caring at Home* (written by Nancy Kohner for the Health Education Authority and the King's Fund, London; published by the National Extension College, 1992). Packed with comprehensive written and tabulated information on statutory and other services, financial and legal matters, time off and coping with day to day problems and feelings. Available from the publishers (tel 01223 358295); price £12.

- *Caring—How to Cope* (written by Janet Horwood; published by the Health Education Authority, 1994). Includes chapters on bereavement and stopping caring. Available from HEA Customer Services (tel 01235 465565); price £4.99.

- Help the Aged (St James's Walk, London EC1 0BE; tel 0171 253 0253) runs Seniorline, a free national information service for older people and their carers—tel 0800 650065 (for hard of hearing callers - Minicom 0800 269626); open 9 am to 4 pm, Monday to Friday.

Specialised information

- *Keeping Fit while Caring* (written by Christine Darby; published by the Family Welfare Association, London, 1984). Available from the association (tel 0171 254 6251) or through public libraries. An account of how to lift, transfer, bathe, etc; details of equipment and keep fit exercises for carers, copiously illustrated with photographs.

- *Link on Lifting* is a two hour video showing techniques for lifting and moving disabled people at home. Available from HopeLine Videos, PO Box 515, London SW15 6LQ; price £19.95 plus £2 postage and packing.

- The Holiday Care Service (2nd floor, Imperial Buildings, Victoria Road, Horley, Surrey RH7 7PZ (tel 01293 774535)) is a charity which provides free information and advice for people with disabilities and their carers. It holds details of accommodation, transport, publications, guides, and sources of financial help for holidays in the United Kingdom and abroad.

- Age Link runs a freephone helpline for carers speaking South Asian languages, covering benefits, statutory and voluntary services—tel 0500 786000.

- The Alzheimer's Disease Society has produced audio tapes about dementia in Hindi, Polish, and Cantonese, with an English translation on every tape. *An Introduction to Dementia* is available from the information section of the society (tel 0171 306 0606); price £3.95.

- *Caring for the Person with Dementia* (written by Chris Lay and Bob Woods; published by the Alzheimer's Disease Society; 3rd edition, 1994) is packed with advice to carers about practical, emotional and financial problems. Available from the Alzheimer's Disease Society (tel 0171 306 0606); price £4 including postage and packing.

- *Safe as Houses—Living Alone with Dementia*. London: Alzheimer's Disease Society, 1994. A resource booklet and personal record card to aid risk management.

- *The 36-Hour Day* (written by N L Mace, P V Rabins, B A Castleton, C Cloke, and E McEwen; published by Hodder and Stoughton; 2nd edition, 1996). A comprehensive account of the nature and practical management of the wide range of problems that carers of people with dementia may need to deal with. There are also chapters on caring for oneself and on residential care. Available from the publisher (tel 0171 873 6000), price £14.99.

- *Caring Together—Guidelines for Carers' Self-Help and Support Groups* (written by Judy Wilson; published by the National Extension College, Cambridge, 1988). Practical advice on starting a group and making it work, including how to find other carers, organise meetings, produce newsletters and press releases, set up a telephone line, and deal with the problems that arise within groups. Now out of print but still available through public libraries.

- *Home Truths* (produced by BBC Radio 2's Social Action Team, 1995) is a booklet, aimed mainly at older people, about elder abuse and how to tackle it. Available for a large self addressed envelope with 31p stamp from Home Truths, PO Box 7, London W5 2GQ.

- The Elder Abuse Response Line, run by Action on Elder Abuse, takes calls from older people, carers, and professionals concerned about elder abuse. It is available on 0800 731 4141 Monday to Friday 10 am to 4.30 pm. It is available in English, Hindi and Gujerati.

Organisations

- *Carers National Association* (20/25 Glasshouse Yard, London EC1A 4JS (tel 0171 490 8818) membership £5 a year) is the principal organisation for people who care for frail, disabled, or ill relatives and friends and for interested professionals. It produces a monthly magazine full of news and information on practical and political issues. It has developed an eight point Carers Code and has launched the campaign for "A Fair Deal for Carers." It has a training unit, running a range of courses for health and social service professionals and voluntary sector workers. In association with Boots the Chemists, the association has produced an eight page booklet entitled *Your guide to getting services*, which is a step by step guide for individual carers to gaining an assessment under the community care legislation of the needs of both the carer and the older person. It has produced a "Carers Emergency Card" for carers to carry so that help will be forthcoming for the cared for person if the carer is suddenly taken ill or has an accident. The association operates an advice line, "Carers Line," between 10 am and noon and 2 pm and 4 pm Monday to Friday—tel 0171 490 8898.

- *Alzheimer's Disease Society* (Gordon House, 10 Greencoat Place, London SW1 1PH (tel 0171 306 0606) no fixed annual subscription) is the main organisation for carers of people with Alzheimer's disease or other dementias and interested professionals. It produces an excellent monthly newsletter that includes regular features on the latest dementia research, good practice in the statutory or voluntary sector, and practical accounts of caring. It has produced a wide range of free information sheets and five freephone numbers for recorded information and advice, including legal and financial information (tel 0800 318771/2/3/4/5). There is a wide network of active local branches, some of which provide services for people with dementia and their carers.

Further reading

Twigg J, Atkin K. *Carers perceived*. Buckingham: Open University Press, 1994. (Includes two fascinating accounts, one of the

influences of feminism, kinship obligation, the New Right, and the disability lobby on the debate about carers, and the other on the role of general practitioners and consultant physicians.)
Parker G, Lawton D. *Different types of care, different types of carer: evidence from the general household survey.* London: HMSO, 1994.
Green H. *General household survey 1985: informal carers.* London: HMSO, 1988.
Brotchie J, Hills D. *Equal shares in caring.* London: Socialist Health Association, 1991.

References

1 Department of Health and Social Services. *Growing older.* London: HMSO, 1981.
2 Goldberg D. *Manual of the general health questionnaire.* Windsor: NFER-Nelson, 1978.
3 Carers National Association. *Who cares? Perceptions of caring and carers.* London: Carers National Association, 1996.
4 Warner N. *Better tomorrows. Report of a national study of carers and the community care changes.* London: Carers National Association, 1995.
5 Department of Health. *Employers and carers.* London: DoH, 1993.
6 House of Commons Social Service Committee. *Community care: carers. Social Service Committee 5th report (1989-90).* London: HMSO, 1990.

13: Community services: health

M PUSHPANGADAN, EILEEN BURNS

Many frail or disabled elderly people are now being maintained in the community, partially at least as a consequence of the Community Care Act 1993. This chapter details the work of the major health professionals who are involved in caring for older people in the community and describes how to access nursing, palliative care, continence, mental health, Hospital at Home, physiotherapy, occupational therapy, equipment, and optical, dental, and dietetic services. In many areas, services are evolving to meet needs and some examples of innovative practice are included.

The provision of health care to elderly people in the community is an important aim of the health service, perhaps particularly since the introduction of the Community Care Act 1993. About 8.5 million people over 65 years old are living in their own homes.[1] Older people comprise 70% of the 6.2 million people with disability, and 92% of elderly disabled people live in their own homes. The general practitioner plays a pivotal role in the delivery and coordination of such patients' health care. This chapter describes the role of other health professionals in caring for older people at home.

Nursing services

After inpatient medical care, rehabilitation and convalescence is often continued and completed in the community. District and liaison nurses provide continuity of care after discharge from hospital.

Liaison nurses are usually employed by hospitals and provide a professional link between hospital and community health services. They can improve the quality of transfer for patients from hospital to the community; liaise with social service departments and help to assess patients' needs; identify and respond to problems occurring at the point of discharge; and improve communication between services.

District nurses provide nursing treatment and support to patients and their caregivers within a variety of community settings— patients' own homes, health centres, and residential homes. They are key people in the community, the vast range of their work includes practical work such as dressing ulcers and pressure sores, maintaining bowel and bladder care and giving injections, as well as supportive components—for example, in palliative care. Referrals for continued nursing care are through general practitioners or through hospital based doctors or nurses. This service has usually been available in the daytime only, but some areas now have a night nursing service.

Specialist nurses provide specific services such as palliative care, continence management, and psychiatric services (see specific subsections below).

Palliative care services

Palliative care is the active total care of patients whose disease no longer responds to curative treatment and for whom the goal must be the best quality of life for them and their families. Most palliative care is for patients with cancer, and well over half the number of patients with advanced cancer are cared for at home by hospice and palliative home care services, which work closely with the patient's general practitioner and primary health care team.

In some areas, Hospice at Home schemes enable patients to stay at home. A comprehensive service, including practical nursing and night sitting, is provided by a multiprofessional team that has access to consultant advice and may be supported by experienced volunteers. The care at home is usually based on Macmillan nurses or the Marie Curie service.

Macmillan nurses were set up by Cancer Relief Macmillan Fund, which itself exists due to Douglas Macmillan who, shocked by the distressing death of his father, set up the charity in 1911 to improve awareness of cancer. The nurses are specially trained to give supportive care and advice and are employed by the NHS. They provide information about illness and treatment and give advice on pain and symptom control and on financial entitlements, such as attendance allowance for caregivers. They offer time to talk through problems and anxieties, provide aids and equipment to assist in care, and provide support to caregivers.

Marie Curie service—The Marie Curie Memorial Foundation

103

was established in 1948 and the name Marie Curie was chosen as a tribute to the scientist who discovered radium. The Marie Curie nurses, of whom there are 5000, provide free "hands on" nursing care for cancer patients in their own homes throughout the day and night; thus they also provide support and respite to informal caregivers. The service usually runs in conjunction with district nursing services, with access through the district nurses or the Marie Curie nurse manager.

Continence services

Urinary incontinence affects 10-20% of elderly women and 7-10% of elderly men living in their own homes, and rates are much higher in elderly people in residential and nursing homes. The consequences of urinary incontinence are both medical and social, with higher rates of depression and social isolation among people who are incontinent. A thorough assessment of all people with incontinence is essential so that appropriate management may be planned. In many places this is provided by a continence service, which aims to promote continence and better management of incontinence and to increase public understanding of incontinence and its management.

The service is usually delivered by a district nurse, who assesses the individual's need. A specialist nurse continence adviser is also usually available, and there may be access to a continence clinic run by a physician, gynaecologist, or urologist with a special interest in the condition. In general the service includes:

- Social and environmental assessment to maintain continence— for example by attention to
  Mobility (walking aids, correct chair height)
  Clothing adaptations (Velcro fasteners, etc)
  Toilet facilities (grab rails, raised toilet seat)
- Advice on fluid intake and diet (encourage adequate fluid intake, reduction of caffeine and alcohol)
- Prevention of constipation
- Bladder retraining
- Pelvic floor muscle exercises
- Help with catheterisation: instruction in self catheterisation and on emptying catheter bags and dealing with blocked catheters
- Counselling for patients and caregivers
- Advice on appropriate aids to deal with incontinence:
  Absorbent products such as pads, pants, and bed protection

Penile sheaths
Commodes and hand held urinals.

In addition, urodynamic studies can be carried out to clarify the mechanism of incontinence. This is especially useful when empirical treatment has failed or when surgery would be clinically appropriate if a correctable condition was found.

Mental health services for elderly people

The elderly mental health services provide an integrated service to older people suffering from either functional or organic mental illness. The service aims to provide prompt assessment, treatment, and rehabilitation of elderly people with mental illness and to maintain them at home wherever possible. Access to the service is usually through general practitioners or other registered medical practitioners. The service is usually organised on a geographical basis. The team, headed by a consultant in old age psychiatry,[2] may include community psychiatric nurses, psychologists, occupational therapists, and physiotherapists.

Community psychiatric nurses offer psychiatric nursing care and monitor the patient's mental state and the effects of psychoactive medication. They may also provide specific treatment such as anxiety management, relaxation techniques, and management of cognitive and behavioural problems.

Clinical psychologists provide psychological evaluation and assessment of cognition, behaviour, mood, and personality. They may contribute to the non-pharmacological management of psychiatric symptoms, such as anxiety or behavioural difficulties.

Occupational therapists and physiotherapists provide assessments and treatment to optimise independence in all activities of daily living.

Some areas have extended home respite schemes, which provide support to patients in their own home, thus reducing the strain on informal caregivers. These serve patients with mental illness, especially dementia.

Hospital at Home

Hospital at Home schemes are still being developed. Starting in 1978 in Peterborough, the first British scheme was based on the

105

Bayonne "hospitalisation à domicile" programme in France. The aim is twofold: to provide a community based scheme which offers medical, nursing, and therapeutic care, support, and treatment to patients in their own homes, either after discharge from hospital or as an alternative to hospital admission; and to improve the quality of discharge from hospital for these patients and to help reduce the length of an inpatient stay.

The team implementing the scheme consists of nursing staff with a named team leader, usually trained in district nursing, who assumes responsibility for assigning health care support workers to the patients and for coordinating the service provision. The team also includes a physiotherapist and an occupational therapist. Patients are referred from hospital wards and from accident and emergency departments, from domiciliary visits by consultants, and from general practitioners and district nurses. Patients are assessed and accepted on to the scheme if their disability is likely to respond to the rehabilitation service of the team and can be managed safely at home (Box 13.1).

Patients are usually supported for a finite period—often four to six weeks. Existing services such as district nursing, social services, day centres, and day hospitals continue to ensure continuity of care, and liaison with these services ensures that there is no duplication in care. The patient is evaluated regularly by the team leader and, when required, by the consultant geriatrician or general practitioner, but a formal review and interdisciplinary assessment of the patient's medical condition and ability to cope with functional activities of daily living is undertaken before discharge. Where appropriate there is handover to statutory services such as home care, meals on wheels, or community physiotherapy. The cost effectiveness of Hospital at Home teams is currently under assessment.

Box 13.1   Suitability for Hospital at Home schemes

- Continued rehabilitation, such as stroke patients
- Patients rendered temporarily dependent—for example, owing to fractures
- Patients who had prolonged hospitalisation and who would benefit from specific rehabilitative programmes in their own homes, to rebuild confidence and restore skills in their own environment

---

Physiotherapy

Community physiotherapists are based in health centres and provide advice, assessment, and short term intervention. They help with problems such as:

- Mobility after a fall, when confidence is reduced
- Mobility after hospitalisation for fractures, hip replacement, etc
- Strokes, giving advice on positioning, handling, and other aspects of rehabilitation
- Giving advice to carers and district nurses on safe handling and lifting
- Dealing with acute musculoskeletal problems
- Giving advice on exercises to prevent muscle wasting.

Referrals are usually through general practitioners, district nurses, consultants, and physiotherapy staff based in hospitals.

Occupational therapy

Community occupational therapists are employed by social services and assess patients in their own homes. Though the main emphasis of their work is in providing equipment, they may be involved in organising extra services such as home help sessions. Occupational therapists may liaise with surveyors and planners regarding major adaptations and advise on the fitting of such items as stair rails, modified toileting and bathing facilities, and stair lifts. The implementation of the Community Care Act has increased demands on this service considerably.

Equipment service

The equipment service provides selected nursing aids and aids to daily living (Box 13.2). These are intended to aid recovery and rehabilitation after illness and to promote the independence of disabled people, to enable them to function in their own home environment.

In many areas there is an arbitrary and illogical distinction between "nursing aids" (supplied by health services, usually free of charge) and "aids to daily living" (supplied by social services, sometimes free). Other agencies are also involved, such as the wheelchair service, which provides specialist seating and wheelchairs, and housing agencies, which provide ramps.

107

Box 13.2   Equipment commonly available from the equipment service

For nursing needs:
- Hoists
- Beds
- Mattresses, including pressure relieving equipment
- Commodes
- Urinals
- Walking sticks and frames

For daily living:
- Raised toilet seats
- Toilet frames
- Bath boards, seats and mats
- Trolleys
- Tap turners
- Grab rails
- Modified cutlery

Patients can get useful advice from disabled living centres (which are run by independent charitable institutions)[3] on what is available[4,5] and where to get it. After the patient has been assessed by an occupational therapist, any health care professional may request equipment from the service.

Skilled assessment is required, so that appropriate aids are safe and effective, and also aesthetically pleasing and acceptable to the patient. The equipment service provides instructions to patients on how to use the device as well as follow up visits to monitor patients' progress.

Optical services

Visual problems become more common with increasing age. Though opticians may now make a charge for an eye test, many people can obtain free NHS sight tests (Box 13.3).

People entitled to free tests may have their sight tested at home if they are unable to get to an optician; they are also entitled to NHS vouchers to help pay for glasses. In addition, war pensioners who require sight tests or glasses as a result of a condition for which they get their pension may be able to claim some or all of the cost from the Department of Social Security.

Box 13.3   Exemption from charges

NHS sight tests
- Registered blind or partially sighted people
- People diagnosed as having diabetes or glaucoma or in a family with glaucoma
- People receiving income support (or whose partner receives income support)
- People with certificate AG2 (qualifying for low income entitlement)
- Patients of hospital ophthalmologists

NHS dental treatment
- People receiving income support (or whose partners receive income support)
- People with certificate AG2

Dental services

Many elderly people retain few natural teeth. It has been estimated that 50% of over 65 year olds in Britain have used a full denture and 30% partial dentures. People who are unable to receive treatment from a general dental practitioner may be treated by the community dental services. Such patients are mainly those with disability or infirmity and also those with medical conditions which make dental treatment more difficult. People who are housebound may be able to get their treatment at home.

The maximum cost of dentistry through the NHS is 80% of most treatments, up to a maximum of £330 for one course of treatment.

Chiropody

Chiropodists restore and maintain foot function and comfort through treatment and health promotion. Four in five people aged 65 or more have at least one foot problem and about half of these need a chiropody service, but it is estimated that only half of these patients currently receive treatment. Chiropody may be provided in community clinics, but domiciliary chiropody is available for patients who are housebound or have poor mobility. Referrals may be made by patients themselves or by doctors and nurses. "At risk" groups, such as people with diabetes, peripheral vascular disease, or peripheral neuropathy, are treated as a priority.

109

Most foot problems fall into the following categories:

- Foot ulcers—these can be neuropathic or ischaemic. In addition to treating foot ulcers, chiropodists give advice on preventive measures such as nail cutting and footwear
- Rheumatoid foot—deformation of the foot can occur by subluxation or dislocation at the metatarsophalangeal joints, and ulceration can occur at sites of nodules and bursae. Chiropodists can advise on appropriate footwear and protective insoles
- Nail problems (ingrowing toenails; onychogryphosis)—elderly people commonly have problems cutting long toenails. This usually arises because of a combination of impaired manual dexterity and limited hip and knee flexion
- Corns—pressure or friction causes these areas of hyperkeratosis; a chiropodist can provide advice on footwear
- Biomechanical problems—chiropodists can manufacture and fit corrective orthoses for mechanical problems of foot structure and function.

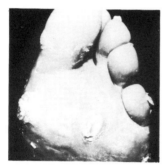 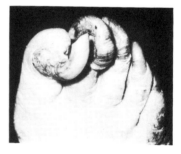

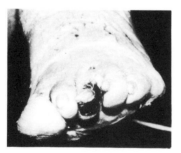

Figure 13.1   Foot problems are common in old age, but can be prevented or ameliorated by chiropody

Chiropody services face a high level of demand. In some areas chiropodists' assistants perform the less technically demanding work. Some older people choose private chiropody, which is usually provided in their home and may be obtained more frequently than chiropody through the NHS.

Nutrition and dietetic services

A medical practitioner can refer an elderly patient at risk of malnutrition (Box 13.4) to a dietitian. The role of dietitians has evolved over the past 20 years, and they now provide nutritional education and treatment in the community. Patients may be seen in day centres, community hospitals, health centres, and at home.

Dietitians may offer simple, practical information about food to allow people to make informed choices about healthy eating or they may offer specific advice to those with particular dietary requirements, such as patients with diabetes or those advised to follow a low fat diet. They may also provide help to patients receiving nasogastric or gastrostomy feeding.

Community pharmacists

As well as running commercial outlets, pharmacists offer advice to patients on the appropriateness of over the counter medications and can advise on risks of adverse drug reactions. Pharmacists may supply drugs dispensed in daily dose reminders,[6] and some will deliver drugs to patients' homes.

Box 13.4   Malnutrition: those at greatest risk

- Age over 75
- Bereaved
- Male
- Living alone
- Housebound
- Suffering from dementia

References

1 *Living in Britain: results from the 1994 general household survey.* London: OPCS, 1994. (Supplement A: people aged 65 and over)
2 Wattis J. What an old age psychiatrist does. *BMJ* 1996;**313**:101-4.
3 Barodawala S. Community care: the independent sector. *BMJ* 1996;**313**:741-3.
4 Mulley GP, ed. *Everyday aids and appliances.* London: BMJ, 1989.
5 Mulley GP, ed. *More everyday aids and appliances.* London: BMJ, 1991.
6 Corlett A. Aids to compliance with medication. *BMJ* (in press).

14: Community care and social services

D RENWICK

The aim of community care is to enable people with various types of disability to live in their own homes, rather than in institutions. This involves the provision of support and services at home by various agencies. After a critical report in 1986 identified problems with coordination and flexibility of community care services, the white paper *Caring for people* (1989) stated the government's aim to provide a "needs led," responsive range of services, promoting maximum independence of those wishing to live at home rather than enter institutional care. New arrangements were introduced in 1993, involving a formal assessment procedure and the production of a personalised care plan for each individual, incorporating services provided by private and voluntary agencies as well as by social services departments. This chapter describes the components of community care services supplied by local social services authorities, including housing adaptations, equipment, telephones and alarms, home care, meals, and respite care.

Before April 1993, social services departments had been involved mainly in the provision of care. With the new community care arrangements, social services became responsible for assessing need, designing care plans, and securing delivery of appropriate services.

To increase the spectrum of care available, social services departments were encouraged to purchase care from private and voluntary agencies, thus becoming "enabling authorities" rather than simply providers of care. In addition, financial support for people in residential or nursing homes also became the responsibility of social services departments.

This chapter describes the community care services supplied by social services departments. Services available from the health authority and from voluntary or private organisations are considered in chapters 12 and 14 in this book. As there is substantial overlap between services provided by these organisations, and as local social services authorities have been encouraged to develop

113

their own arrangements for the provision of community care, organisations providing particular services may vary in different parts of the country.

Entry to the system: the role of the social worker

For both doctors and patients, the key figure in access to community care services is the social worker, who may be based in a hospital medical department for care of elderly patients or old age psychiatry, in a general practice or health centre, or in the local social services office. Social workers will accept referrals from any source, have information on all services available locally, and act as a liaison between the various agencies involved in the provision of care. The management of less complex problems (for example, a request for home care only) may be undertaken by a social welfare officer, social work assistant, or social services care manager rather than a social worker.

When an individual who may need extra support at home is referred, the social worker will usually start a formal assessment procedure. The complexity of the assessment process varies from an initial assessment of mobility, personal care abilities, current environment, and support network to a more comprehensive process involving input from other members of the interdisciplinary team (including medical staff) and including assessment of finances.

Residential and nursing homes

Social services departments are responsible for the provision of local authority residential homes, sometimes called aged persons homes or part III homes or, in Scotland, part IV homes. Private residential homes must be registered with the local social services department; the social services inspection and monitoring unit visits them regularly to ensure that standards are maintained (the health authority is responsible for inspecting private nursing homes). Lists of registered private residential and nursing homes are held by social workers in the area. Chapter 10 gives further information about homes for elderly people.

When a comprehensive assessment indicates the need for care in a nursing or residential home, a financial assessment will be performed by social services to identify whether assistance with funding will be offered.

Housing adaptations

Each social services office has a disability services team made up of community occupational therapists, social workers specialising in physical disability, and rehabilitation officers for visually impaired people. The team deals with applications for home adaptations, including stair lifts or rails, grab rails, bathroom adaptations, widening doors for wheelchairs, siting of sockets or switches in convenient positions, and extra heating appliances.

These adaptations will be provided by the social services department if the applicant is physically or mentally disabled or has sensory impairment and if independence or care at home cannot continue, or the applicant will be potentially at risk, without the adaptation. A community occupational therapist will perform a home visit to assess whether the application is appropriate; eligibility for funding will be determined by a financial assessment by social services (Box 14.1). For major adaptations, a survey by an environmental health officer may be necessary before approval by the housing department.

Equipment for daily living

The community occupational therapist can give advice on, assess the need for, and arrange provision of various types of equipment to promote safety and independence in dressing, personal hygiene, using the toilet, cooking and domestic activities, and reaching and lifting. Equipment will be provided if the applicant is physically or mentally disabled, or has sensory impairment, and if assessment indicates that equipment is necessary for maintaining independence or care at home. Separate criteria may exist for the provision

---

Box 14.1 Funding for adaptations to housing for elderly people

- Applications for housing adaptations are assessed by the disability services team
- Minor adaptations may be provided free of charge to suitable applicants by the social services department
- Major adaptations to council housing will be funded by the housing department; in some areas tenants may be expected to contribute to the cost
- Private home owners undergo a financial assessment and may be expected to meet a proportion of the costs

---

of items such as specialised seating, bath lifts, and showers.

Provision of mobility aids (walking sticks and frames) is the responsibility of the health authority and may require assessment by a community physiotherapist. Wheelchairs are provided by the district wheelchair service after assessment by an occupational therapist.

Equipment is usually provided free of charge on permanent loan. Maintenance and repair of equipment and adaptations is generally the responsibility of the user, even when equipment has been supplied by the social services department.

Equipment for nursing needs (mattresses, beds, etc) is supplied by the health authority. What is considered as equipment for daily living and what is deemed nursing equipment varies from area to area.

Telephones

In certain circumstances, social services departments will contribute to the cost of telephone installation and rental charges (Box 14.2).

Special telephone adaptations and equipment are also available from the social services department for people who are unable to use a standard telephone because of disability:

- Partial hearing loss—incoming speech amplifier; volume and pitch control
- Profound deafness—special telephone set
- Sight impairment—large dial ring or buttons; memory buttons
- Inability to hold the handset—"hands free" telephone
- Speech impairment or weak voice—outgoing speech amplifier or

---

Box 14.2 Eligibility for funding for telephone installation and rental

- Physical or mental disability or sensory impairment
- Receiving financial support (income support, housing benefit, etc)
- Living alone or with a carer who could not be expected to deal with an emergency
- At risk unless able to contact helpers in an emergency

---

speech synthesiser.

The disability services team at the local social services office arranges provision of these specially adapted telephones.

Emergency alarm systems

In general, 24 hour emergency call systems consist of a press button and loudspeaker installed in the home or a portable pendant button that is worn round the neck or as a bracelet or brooch. A central control centre will contact a nominated carer or the emergency services if the alarm is triggered. Social services departments may provide such systems for people who are elderly or disabled; living alone or with a carer who could not be expected to deal with an emergency; at risk if unable to contact helpers in an emergency; unable to use an ordinary or adapted telephone; or at risk of recurrent falls or collapses.

Applications are assessed by the disability services team. After the financial assessment, a contribution to the cost of the system may be requested.

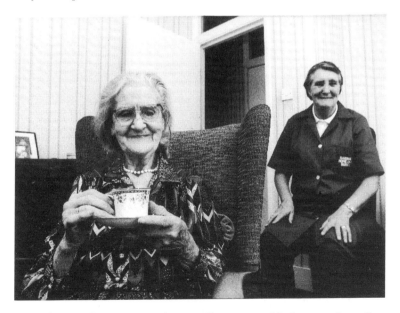

Figure 14.1 Home care services can improve an elderly person's quality of life. Reproduced courtesy of Ulrike Preuss.

Home care

Previously expected only to help with housework and shopping, home care workers ("home helps") now also contribute to aspects of personal care (getting into or out of bed, dressing, washing, toileting) as well as with household tasks, laundry, shopping, and collecting prescriptions or pensions. There is some overlap with the role of community nurses, and responsibility for bathing clients or overseeing medication may vary locally.

Applications for home care are dealt with by the home care manager, who can be contacted through the local social services office. An assessment visit will be performed to determine what input is required, and then a health care worker will be allocated for a number of visits per day or hours per week. The service is available during the daytime seven days a week.

After a financial assessment, a charge is made for the service, and this may vary locally. In some cases, therefore, it is cheaper for the older person to arrange for private help; this also avoids being means tested.

Nursing or supportive care during the night is not provided by social services agencies. Where this is included in a care plan, it will be purchased from a private agency. A financial contribution towards the cost of this may be requested.

Meals

Social services departments organise schemes to provide a midday meal to people who are elderly or disabled, are house-bound, have no help with shopping or cooking, or would otherwise lack adequate nutrition. These meals are available at low cost, and special diets can be catered for.

Meals on wheels—This service delivers a hot cooked meal to the home once daily, up to seven days a week. There is a fixed charge per meal.

Frozen meals—To allow more flexibility, bulk deliveries of precooked frozen meals are also available, with the loan of a freezer for clients who do not own one. Charges are similar to those for meals on wheels.

Intermittent ("respite") care

Intermittent care aims to ease the pressure on informal carers by substituting an alternative method of care for a period of time—a few hours, a few days, or several weeks. It may be arranged on a "one off" basis or as a regular standing arrangement, for example for two weeks in every two months.

Sitting service—In some areas, social services departments run schemes where volunteers will "sit" with an elderly person in his or her own home. This provides companionship for elderly people living alone, or gives the carer a break. This service is usually free of charge, although the volunteers will have travel expenses reimbursed.

Day centres may be run by social services or by voluntary organisations. Attendance on one or more days a week provides a break for carers and also support for vulnerable elderly people living alone. Transport and lunch are provided at a small charge. Some day centres have days especially devoted to the care of people with dementia, people of particular ethnic groups, or people with sensory impairment.

Family placement schemes—Many social services departments hold lists of local families who have volunteered to offer intermittent care for an elderly person. Attempts are made to "match" each client with an appropriate household. A fixed weekly charge is made to the client; the family receives a small payment. This allows people to enjoy a break in a domestic setting rather than have respite in a home.

Intermittent care in residential or nursing home—Intermittent care may be arranged in either a local authority residential home or a private residential or nursing home. Some homes have dedicated beds for intermittent care; in others, availability of beds may be a problem. Some offer fixed in-out regimens rather than considering individual needs. Local social services departments may have a "bed bureau" to help in the search for a bed. A fixed charge is payable for local authority homes; social services may meet a proportion of the cost of intermittent care in a private home, after financial assessment.

"Holidays"—In some areas, social services departments have arrangements with local authority homes in different regions (for example, in a seaside resort) to allow a period of care to be taken as a holiday.

For people who have complex disability or multiple medical problems, care at a day hospital or in a hospital bed might be more appropriate than care in their own home or a residential home. This can be arranged by the local hospital department of elderly medicine after referral by a general practitioner (Box 14.3).

119

Box 14.3   Types of intermittent care provided by social services departments

- Sitting service
- Day centre attendance
- Family placement schemes
- Respite care in residential or nursing home

Services for elderly people with sensory impairment

Local social services departments hold a register of blind and partially sighted people. Registration is voluntary, and follows referral to and examination by an ophthalmologist.

Rehabilitation officers for visually handicapped people work as members of the disability services team and can give advice to help a person with impaired vision cope with the activities of daily living. This may include training in communication methods and techniques to improve mobility, and special equipment (for example clocks, telephones) may be provided.

Social services rehabilitation officers also act as a link with voluntary services for visually impaired or deaf people. Social services departments or voluntary bodies may run day centres for partially sighted or blind people and deaf people; local authority homes that specialise in the care of visually impaired people are found in some areas.

Further reading

Mandelstam M. *How to get equipment for disability*. London: Jessica Kingsley and Kogan Page for the Disabled Living Foundation; third edition, 1996.

Groves T, ed. *Countdown to community care*. London: BMJ Publishing, 1993.

Meredith B. *The community care handbook. The reformed system explained*. London: Age Concern England; second edition, 1995.

15: Community care: the independent sector

S BARODAWALA

The independent sector, which consists of the voluntary and private sectors, is a vital element in supporting older people in the community. The voluntary sector, coordinated by the Council for Voluntary Service and the National Council for Voluntary Organisations, provides a variety of services, including practical help, reassurance and companionship, and advice, information, campaigning, and advocacy. The private sector owns all of the nursing homes and most of the residential homes and is gradually becoming more involved with the provision of services to help support older people in their own homes. With this increase in size and importance of the independent sector over recent years, there is now a real need for greater communication between the private, voluntary, and statutory agencies in any one region. In some areas, forums made up of representatives of these various sectors meet to discuss relevant issues and construct local policies, thus allowing a more coordinated approach to the delivery of services.

Over the past 20 years the emphasis on supporting older people has shifted from institutional care to care in the community, which is provided in combination by the social services department, the voluntary and private sectors, and informal groups.

Since the implementation of the Community Care Act in 1993, the needs of older people and their carers are now formally assessed; ideally, suitable services are then provided. These reforms have meant that voluntary and private organisations are now increasingly being asked to provide residential care, day care, and home based services under contract to social services departments.

The voluntary sector

The role of the voluntary sector in society is becoming ever more important. Voluntary organisations vary tremendously from large, national organisations with paid staff, to small, local charities providing advocacy, self help, and specific services to communities. Also, as needs and resources differ regionally, the services available vary from locality to locality. Despite this diversity, all voluntary groups share the philosophy that no person should suffer oppression or lack of opportunity because of race, gender, belief, sexuality, disability, age, class, or geographical location, and that local voluntary and community action is a means of combating disadvantage and contributes to the quality of life for groups, communities, and individuals in local areas.

Coordinating voluntary organisations

As the role of the voluntary sector in society grows and becomes ever more complex, it no longer makes sense for the voluntary organisations to work in isolation. Two organisations work with voluntary groups, at national and local levels, providing help and support and promoting their work (Box 15.1). They also provide a vital link with the statutory authorities, which is important for planning services in a specific area.

Council for Voluntary Service—The CVS is itself a voluntary organisation. It works with other voluntary groups in a local area, helping to coordinate the existing services they provide and to develop new services as required. It also provides information to the general public, health professionals, statutory departments, and other voluntary organisations. Local branches are given in the Yellow Pages or can be obtained from the National Association of Councils for Voluntary Service.

National Council for Voluntary Organisations—The NCVO is the representative body for the voluntary sector in England. It brings voluntary organisations together so that they can work together, learn from each other, maximise scarce resources, and make their voice heard.

Box 15.1 Addresses of national organisations

National Association of Councils for Voluntary Service (NACVS), 3rd floor, Arundel Court, 177 Arundel Street, Sheffield S1 2NU (tel 0114 278 6636)
National Council for Voluntary Organisations, Regents Wharf, 8 All Saints Street, London N1 9RL (tel 0171 713 6161)

Box 15.2   Addresses of blanket organisations

Age Concern England, Astral House, 1268 London Road, London
SW16 4ER (tel 0181 679 8000)
Help the Aged, St James's Walk, Clerkenwell Green, London EC1R
0BE (tel 0171 253 0253)

Blanket organisations

Some voluntary organisations—such as Age Concern and Help
the Aged—are concerned with the overall issues of old age (Box
15.2). They campaign for the interests of older people, research
into their needs, and provide local and national services to help
elderly people. They have also become important in raising public
awareness of the challenges of aging and in furthering educational
activities.

Age Concern has been working for over 50 years to ensure that
older people get the support, encouragement, and care they
require. This is achieved through a network of 100 national
organisations and over 1400 local Age Concern schemes. The
schemes provide practical help at a local level in the form of day
centres, hospital aftercare, advocacy, and insurance schemes. Age
Concern England supports this work through fund raising,
training, campaigning, research, the provision of information, and
publishing.

Help the Aged works to improve the quality of life of older people
in the United Kingdom and internationally. It does this through
information provision; fund raising and campaigning for the rights
of older people; practical help at a local level, such as the provision
of day centres, community transport, home safety, and community
alarms; and its free national information service, Senior Line (tel
0800 289404).

Specific organisations

Disabilities associated with old age (Box 15.3)

The Alzheimer's Disease Society was founded to give advice and
support to those looking after someone with any form of dementia.
There are over 200 local branches and support groups. The society
also promotes research into the disease and lobbies at national and
local level on the behalf of sufferers and their carers.

123

Box 15.3   Addresses of disability related organisations

Alzheimer's Disease Society, Gordon House, 10 Greencoat Place, London SW1P 1PH (tel 0171 306 0606)
Stroke Association, Whitecross Street, London EC1Y 8JJ (tel 0171 490 7999)
Parkinson's Disease Society, 22 Upper Woburn Place, London WC1H 0RA (tel 0171 388 5798)
Arthritis Care, 18 Stephenson's Way, London NW1 2HD (tel 0171 916 1500)
Royal National Institute for the Blind (RNIB), 224 Great Portland Street, London W1N 6AA (tel 0171 388 1266)
Royal National Institute for Deaf People (RNID), 19-23 Featherstone Street, London EC1Y 8FL (tel 0171 296 8000)
Royal Association for Disability and Rehabilitation (RADAR), 12 City Forum, 250 City Road, London EC1V 8AF (tel 0171 250 3222)
Disablement Information and Advice Line (DIAL UK), Park Lodge, St Catherine's Hospital, Tick Hill Road, Doncaster DN4 8QN (tel 01302 310123)

The Stroke Association, together with its Scottish sister organisation, The Chest, Heart and Stroke Association, is concerned with stroke victims and their families. It promotes research, health education, rehabilitation, and advisory and welfare services. The Stroke Association Volunteer Service provides home visiting and group meetings; its main aim is to help dysphasic stroke patients attain maximum possible recovery and become as independent as possible. The Stroke Family Support Service is a visiting service for all stroke victims, and it can refer patients to more specialised sources, such as a disabled living centre, other voluntary agencies, or local stroke clubs. Referrals to the support service can be made via hospital, the general practitioner, a social worker, or by self referral.

The Parkinson's Disease Society has more than 200 local branches. Nationally, most of its work consists of information provision, medical research, and promoting the welfare of patients with Parkinson's disease. The local branches offer opportunities for mutual support, social activities, fund raising, and practical help.

Arthritis Care is the British national welfare organisation for sufferers from arthritis. It aims to help sufferers by providing information, advice, and practical aid. Arthritis Care also has

124

holiday centres equipped with ramps, rails, and many other facilities to increase the independence and enjoyment of disabled people.

The Royal National Institute for the Blind (RNIB) is a large organisation providing help and guidance to people who are registered as blind or partially sighted. Currently, 1 in 7 of people aged 75 and over is blind or partially sighted. It has a talking book service, a weekly newspaper—*Big Print*—a housing advisory service, leisure activities, residential care, and hotels. Products to help with everyday living, such as easy to see watches and clocks, kitchen equipment, and white canes, are available by post.

The Royal National Institute for Deaf People (RNID) represents deaf, hard of hearing, and deaf-blind people. Its services include information, residential care, a tinnitus help line, and providing helpful devices such as TV listening devices, flashing doorbells, and alarm clocks. The national telephone relay service, Typetalk, enables deaf people to communicate with hearing people over the telephone network.

The Royal Association for Disability and Rehabilitation (RADAR) offers advice and assistance on a variety of issues affecting people with physical disabilities—housing, aids and adaptations, access, and holidays and leisure.

The Disablement Information and Advice Line (DIAL UK) provides information and advice on a wide range of issues affecting people with disabilities and their carers.

Disabled living centres provide education and information to disabled people who require technical aids. There are more than 20 such centres around Britain. Visitors are given advice on equipment and the opportunity to try it out, costings, and details of where aids can be obtained. The address of the nearest centre can be obtained from DIAL UK.

Organisations for carers

Only in recent years have voluntary organisations and social service departments begun to consider the needs of carers in planning provision. Currently, over six million people in the United Kingdom are looking after a disabled friend or relative at home. Doing this day in, day out can cause tremendous stress, particularly if the whole burden of responsibility falls on the carer. In these circumstances carers frequently feel isolated or become ill. There are several organisations whose primary aim is to provide practical help to caregivers (Box 15.4).

Box 15.4 Addresses of organisations for carers

Crossroads Scheme, 3rd Floor, Dilke House, Malet Street, London
WC1E 7JA (tel 0171 637 1855)
Carers National Association, 20/25 Glasshouse Yard, London EC1A
4JS (carers helpline: tel 0171 490 8898)

Crossroads—The Crossroads organisation began in 1974. There
are over 200 branches nationwide in the UK. The schemes are
developed in partnership with local health and social services
departments to ensure that they complement existing services.
Crossroads services are tailored to meet the needs of the individual
carer and family: each trained care attendant takes over the role of
the main family carer in the home setting. Crossroads also provides
respite care, carer support groups, and a carer helpline. The service
is available 24 hours a day and 365 days a year.

The Carers National Association is another large organisation
providing help and advice for carers. It produces a monthly
magazine and has a training unit as well as other services.[1]

Associations with local focus

Organisations with a local focus are extremely valuable within
each community. Their telephone numbers can be obtained from
the Yellow Pages or the local branch of the Council for Voluntary
Service.

- Women's Royal Voluntary Service (WRVS)
- Citizens' Advice Bureaux
- Neighbourhood schemes
- Community based day centres and luncheon clubs.

Organisations with cultural or religious themes

With the increase in numbers of elderly people from ethnic
minorities living in British communities, there is a great need for
organisations to provide the specialised care and support they
require.

- Jewish Welfare Board
- Asian People with Disabilities Alliance
- Black Elders Associations.

Other services available through the voluntary sector

Gardening and other jobs around the house—Some of the smaller, more locally based voluntary organisations may be able to provide services such as gardening and decorating for older people who are not able to do these tasks themselves. They usually charge only for materials used. Details may be available from the local Council for Voluntary Service.

Domiciliary visiting schemes—Many organisations run visiting schemes whose main aim is to alleviate the loneliness and social isolation of older people—for example, Age Concern run a "Friendly Visitor" scheme.

Transport—Many older people are unable to use public transport as a result of age, disability, or ill health. Some voluntary organisations such as the WRVS, British Red Cross, St John Ambulance, Help the Aged, and Age Concern have wheelchair accessible transport to take members on outings and to and from day centres or hospital. A minimal fee to cover petrol costs may be charged, and on occasions the organisations may actually hire out their vehicles. Some organisations have a pool of volunteer drivers who use their own cars to transport older people to and from their destinations. In certain areas the British Red Cross and St John Ambulance are able to provide an ambulance with an escort for a minimal fee to cover costs—this varies from area to area. Dial-a-ride runs a door to door bus service for the benefit of older people and anyone with a disability; its vehicles are also available for community groups.

Holiday schemes—Information about holidays for older and disabled people can be obtained from the Holiday Care Service free of charge. It can provide advice and possible suggestions for people with special needs but does not actually arrange or book the holidays. Several charities organise their own holidays, some for more active older people and others for more frail or disabled people. Some charities have their own suitably adapted holiday homes or hotels; others (Age Concern, the RNIB, the RNID,

---

Box 15.5   Useful addresses

Holiday Care Service, 2nd Floor, Imperial Buildings, Victoria Road, Horley, Surrey RH6 7PZ (tel 01293 774535)
WRVS National Office, Milton Hill House, Milton Hill, Abingdon, Oxfordshire OX13 6AF (tel 01235 442900)

Arthritis Care, Parkinson's Disease Society) organise group holidays for those of similar interests. Some charities may give grants towards holidays, and information on all these points can be obtained from the Holiday Care Service or the voluntary organisation in question.

Housing associations are non-profit making bodies, run by voluntary committees, providing housing and associated amenities, such as wardens, provision of meals, or homecare. Examples include national schemes such as Anchor Housing, Chantry Housing, and Help the Aged Housing Association. There are also local schemes and schemes aimed at particular groups, such as the British Legion Housing Association.

Hospices—Services provided through the hospice movement include:

- Inpatient units providing symptom control, respite care, and continuing care for terminally ill patients
- Homecare services and domiciliary nursing services to provide assistance for patients and carers in their own homes

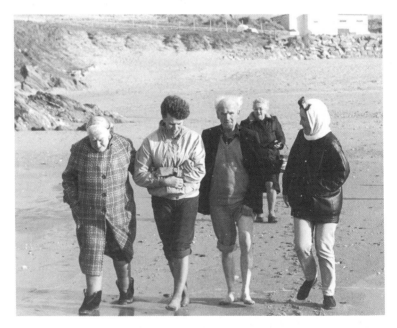

Figure 15.1 Several charities organise holidays for older or disabled people, or give grants for holidays; the Holiday Care Service coordinates such information for disabled or disadvantaged people.

• A bereavement service for relatives and families. Referral to the hospice is usually made by the hospital or general practitioner.

The private sector

In the 1980s the private sector rapidly grew to become the main supplier of nursing homes and residential care. After the Community Care Act was implemented in 1993, this growth slowed down, and the focus has changed to provide more services for those wishing to remain in their own homes. A wide range of services can be available through the private sector, but for a person to be funded by the social services department, the provision of such services is subject to an assessment of need and an assessment of financial resources (Chapter 10). Anyone may purchase these services using their own finances, but this can be prohibitively expensive. All nursing homes and some residential homes are privately owned. If a person is eligible for community care funding, the social services will provide a set amount towards the cost. This may or may not cover complete costs, depending on the particular home.

The private sector can also provide:

• Homecare services to provide help with tasks such as cooking, cleaning, washing, dressing and shopping
• A "night sleeper" service for those who need reassurance or supervision overnight
• Live-in companions, to provide constant care and comfort on a long or short term basis
• 24 hour helplines—in the event of an emergency such as a fall, a press on the alert button on the telephone or on a pendant or bracelet alarm results in an immediate response from trained staff at a central control centre (some social services departments also provide this service)
• Domiciliary nursing services—trained nursing supervision can be provided up to 24 hours a day and 365 days a year. This may be more expensive than care in a nursing home, so if the person is funded by social services his or her choice may be overridden by financial considerations.

The telephone numbers of the private organisations providing these services can be obtained from the Yellow Pages under headings such as Nurses' agencies and care agencies, Nursing homes, and Disabled—information and equipment. Social workers may also be able to provide detailed information on this subject.

Reference

Travers A. Caring for older people: carers. *BMJ* 1996;**313**:482-6.

Index

WITHDRAWN
FROM STOCK
QMUL LIBRARY